CW01676792

AURAL CARE
Protocols and Guidelines

By

Tristram Lesser *MS FRCS*
Consultant Otolaryngologist

Janet Robinson *RGN*
Nurse Practitioner, Southport General Infirmary

Sponsored by – Options Medical Limited and Exmoor Plastics Limited

Published by: Options Medical Limited
16 Katana House, Fort Fareham, Newgate Lane, Fareham, Hampshire PO14 1AH

Copyright © Tristram Lesser & Janet Robinson, 2009
Second Edition

All rights reserved.

No part of this publication may be reproduced, stored in a retrieval system, or transmitted, in any form or by any means, without the prior permission in writing of the publisher, nor be otherwise circulated in any form of binding or cover other than that in which it is published and without a similar condition including this condition being imposed on the subsequent purchaser.

ISBN: 978-0-9555483-1-4

INDEX

Introduction

This second edition of Aural Care is produced at a time when nurse led microsuction aural care clinics are the standard in care. It describes the conditions treated and the criteria for training and the targets for the training of nurses. It gives an example training programme and advice on setting up and running a microsuction clinic. As there is a need for integrated care between the primary care setting where most wax removal is done, we provide the evidence-based guidelines for the management of wax. This allows the place of aural care clinics to be seen in context, as it gives evidence as to what should be done for the patients prior to referral for these conditions. The protocols for aural microsuction, removal of wax, treatment of otitis externa, care of mastoid cavities, furuncle treatment and removal of foreign body as well as administration of aural medications are provided. Audits from one such clinic are detailed and it is important to remember that all such clinics need to be regularly audited. There are a few case studies to provide examples of prescribing for the ear and tables to be used for training.

NURSE-LED AURAL CARE

The UKCC published new regulations in July 1992 which were designed to free the profession from the previous rules that limited nurses to basic, traditional duties. This new freedom led to the development of such roles as Nurse Practitioner and Clinical Nurse Specialists, roles requiring a high level of knowledge, expertise and practical ability in circumscribed, specialised areas.

E.N.T out-patients nurses have taken advantage of these developments and opportunities available to expand their role and to compliment the work of the doctors in many areas. Nurse led Aural care is important and exciting clinical role. Aural care has been performed in the past by nurses using direct vision and dry mopping techniques. Micro-suction is however, the best available method of aural toilet for patients with many acute and chronic ear conditions.

Whilst nurses need to be accountable for their actions and only undertake care for which they feel adequately prepared, there are some formal, validated training courses in aural care. The development of the role should be under the direct supervision of the Consultant in charge, who will ultimately take full responsibility for the treatments that the nurse gives. There are also basic issues that need to be considered before any training is undertaken

- Education
- Accountability
- Support
- Motivation
- Assessment

NURSE PRESCRIBING

An aural care clinic cannot function as nurse-led unless the nurse is able to provide the medications necessary to treat the patient. The issues surrounding nurse prescribing are many and protracted, however group protocols allow the nurse to supply and administer medications to patients who are not individually named but have the condition specified in the protocol.

A group protocol is a specific instruction for the supply and administration of a named medication in a named clinical situation. Protocols should be drawn up by a multidisciplinary team of doctors, pharmacists, nurses and managers.

Local requirements for protocols should be adhered to but there are basic requirements central to all.

- Description of the medication
- The clinical condition the protocol applies to
- Detailed information on dosage, form, route, frequency and duration of administration
- Contra-indications and side effects
- Who can administer the medication
- Signatures of the doctor, pharmacist and manager
- Date the protocol was written and is due for review
- How records are to be kept and audited

EAR PROBLEMS COMMONLY SEEN

EXTERNAL EAR CONDITIONS

EAR WAX

Epithelial migration

Body skin is constantly shed, usually as a result of friction from clothing or washing. This is not possible in the ear as it would just fill up so it has developed migration. All the skin starts growing at the centre of the tympanic membrane and migrates to the edges of the ear drum where it continues laterally. When it reaches the hair-bearing outer part of the canal the superficial layers separate. The skin then mixes with the secretion of the ceruminous and sebaceous glands to form ear wax. The glands are found in the skin of the outer third of the external acoustic meatus and secrete a liquid material at the base of the hairs. After secretion, evaporation occurs to leave a sticky, waxy substance that is able to trap dirt.

WAX

Wax comes in one of two forms, wet and dry. Wet wax is produced by most African and Caucasians and is moist, sticky and honey-coloured. Dry wax is more common in Mongoloid ethnic groups and tends to be greyer in colour, less sticky, granular and flakey. The gene for wet wax is dominant. Ear wax tends to become drier and harder with age. Wax is normally loosened by transmission of movement from the temporomandibular joint from chewing or talking, allowing its passage out of the ear. This natural process can be upset by a number of factors and cause wax impaction. Impaction is commoner in males owing to the presence of thicker, coarser hairs in the lateral part of the ear. Narrow canals, use of cotton buds and even a hearing aid mould may impede the normal flow of wax. Sometimes no obvious cause is found to account for the impaction.

Clinical Features

Impaction of wax can cause a blocked feeling, deafness, pain, dizziness, itching, noises and occasionally coughing (via the auricular branch of the vagus nerve, called Arnolds nerve), this is also why some people cough when they ear is cleaned. These symptoms are improved by removing the wax.

Management

Syringing involves the use of a metal or electric pump syringe. These direct a jet of warm (body temperature) water along the roof or posterior canal wall so that it passes behind the wax and forces it outwards. The procedure is often preceded by drops (sodium bicarbonate drops are efficacious, safe and inexpensive). Although relatively safe, complications may occur and include coughing, pain, local trauma, otitis externa and rarely tympanic membrane perforation. Contraindications to syringing are listed in detail below. In such cases removal under direct vision with microscope using microsuction or wax hooks is a more appropriate and safer alternative.

KERATOSIS OBTURANS

This uncommon condition occurs when there is a failure of the normal skin migration. Debris collect in the deep part of the external auditory meatus. As with collections of keratin anywhere, this sets up a low-grade inflammatory response resulting in a re-absorption of bone and widening of the bony canal.

Clinical Features

Patients usually present with an acute exacerbation of the inflammatory process. Pain is usually the dominant feature, although there is inevitably a hearing loss from the occluded canal. The appearances are similar to an acute otitis externa around impacted wax. The keratin takes this appearance because the part in contact with the air oxidizes and changes colour.

Management

Removal of the keratin plug is essential to control the inflammatory process. This is often difficult as the patient is usually in considerable pain and a general anaesthetic required. Topical antibiotic/steroid combinations are used to treat the secondary otitis externa. In the long term these patients require periodic aural toilet.

EXOSTOSES AND OSTEOMAS

Osteomas are uncommon benign round tumours of bone usually arising from the ear canal. Exostoses, on the other hand, are common. They are hyperostoses of the tympanic bone of the external canal and probably caused by a periosteal reaction to exposure to cold, usually from swimming. In both conditions, although the lumen of the canal is reduced, they rarely result in symptoms. If problems do occur they are usually related to impairment of the normal process of epithelial migration. In these cases surgical removal may be indicated. Osteomas can often be removed via the external canal, while exostoses will more often require a formal postaural or endaural approach. They are easy to diagnosis as they are bony hard and hurt if prodded to hard.

FOREIGN BODIES IN THE EAR

Foreign bodies are put into the ears more commonly by school children than by toddlers. The objects can be organic (pieces of paper, rubber, pencil, seeds, peas and beans) or inorganic (beads, buttons, crayons and stones). Inorganic foreign bodies are often asymptomatic, but organic objects may give rise to otitis externa by local irritation. One of the most common cause of this is cotton wool, and it is not unusual to find this in adult patients who have been attempting to clean their ears. Less common are, but more irritating, insects, either dead or dying.

Management

A foreign body in the external ear canal is usually seen on otoscopy. Removal may appear to be easy, but usually requires the skills and the facilities of a specialist, or ENT doctor. Ill-directed attempts at their removal by the untrained may lead to complications. It is sometimes possible to remove the foreign body in the clinic, but a general anaesthetic may be required for children and sensitive adults.

Treatment

Many foreign bodies can be removed by syringing. Objects of vegetable origin, such as peas, beans and nuts, may swell and should not be syringed. Large objects lying superficial to the external ear canal isthmus should not be syringed as there is a danger of wedging them in that area.

Suction or a fine hook, with the object viewed with an operating microscope is needed to remove material of vegetable origin and large objects which lie superficial too the isthmus.

Forceps are useful for soft material such as paper, cotton wool or sponge but should never be used to remove smooth spherical objects such as beads, as they will tend to push them further down the ear canal.
Insects should be killed before syringing by instilling spirit drops into the ear canal. Maggots grip on the external ear-canal skin, so must be killed or anaesthetises with chloroform water prior to syringing.

Once the object is out, the tympanic membrane should be examined to ensure it has not been damaged. If there is an otitis externa a swab should be taken, the ear cleaned and antibiotic-steroid ear drops instilled.

OTITIS EXTERNA

Definition

Otitis externa is defined as inflammation of the skin of the external auditory canal (EAC).

Pathology

The skin of the EAC has in the outer third an epithelial layer containing hair follicles, ceruminous glands and sebaceous glands, over a thin dermal layer containing sweat glands. This skin of the bony ear canal lacks these and is verythin and tightly bound to the bone. The secretions of the sebaceous glands keep the skin watertight and supple. Sweat gland secretions are acidic and keep the secretion at a pH between three and five which is lethal for most human pathogens. Usually the EAM contains Staphylococcus albus and other commensals which can include pseudomonas organisms in small amounts.

In acute phase of otitis externa there are dilated dermal blood vessels of increased permeability which cause signs of a red, hot, oedematous and tender ear canal.

Predisposing factors

- Heat, humidity, bathing, swimming
- Trauma, especially from dirty fingernails, cotton buds and hairgrips
- Inherited – narrow ear canals and certain blood types
- Dermatological conditions such as proriasis, eczema and seborrhoeic dermatitis

Classification

1. *Infective*

a) **Bacterial**

Diffuse otitis externa commonly caused by *Pseudomonas aeruginosa, S. aureus* and *Proteus*.
Furunculosis, usually caused by *S. aureus.*
Necrotising otitis externa, usually caused by *P. aeruginosa* or occasionally *S. aureus.*
Erysipelas caused *by Streptococcus pyogenes.*
Perichondritis.
Otitis media.

b) **Fungal**

Aspergillus niger
Aspergillus fumigatus
Candida albicans

c) **Viral**

Herpes simplex
Herpes Zoster (Ramsey Hunt Syndrome)
Presumptive in bullous haemorrhagica

2. **Reactive**

Eczema
Seborrhoeic dermatitis
Allergy to drops
Keratosis obturans
Psoriasis
Dandruff

Clinical Features

Otitis externa may be confined to the meatus (localized) or involve other areas of skin (generalized). Localised infection can be circumscribed or diffuse while generalized infection can be either primary otological or primarily dermatological.

Ask about direct trauma to the ear canal, swimming habits, atopic tendency and previous otological problems. Symptoms of infection elsewhere and preceding otitis media should also be sought.

The history may provide a pointer towards the diagnosis, severe itching suggests eczema, allergy or mycotic infection. Pain occurs with furunculosis, diffuse otitis externa and herpes infections.

On examination erythema is a feature of eczema, seborrhoeic dermatitis, mycosis or acute trauma. Vesicles occur in eczema,and herpatic infection, excess squamous debris suggests chronic eczema or mycosis and hypertrophic meatal skin suggest chronic disease.

It is not uncommon to find the ear canal closed by swelling in a patient with acute otalgia. A careful examination will usually distinguish furunculosis (common) from acute mastoiditis (now much less common). In the former there may be post-aural tenderness localized to a palpable lymph node. Exceptionally this node may break down to cause diffuse tenderness and oedema which may displace the pinna slightly forwards and there is always pain on moving the pinna. A patient with acute mastoiditis will have a more marked post-aural swelling which may be fluctuant, displacing the pinna down as well as forwards. There is less pain on moving the pinna and there will be a preceding history of acute suppurative otitis media.

Investigations

A culture swab should be taken for microbiological culture, including fungal culture, and antibiotic/antimycotic sensitivity.

Management

1. Meticulous and if needed repeated aural toilet, paying particular attention to the antero-inferior meatal recess.

2. Splinting open the meatus. The two recommended choices are 12 millimetre ribbon gauze, impregnanted with 10% Ichthammol in Glycerine, the hydroscopic action of which reduces meatál swelling or a Pope's sponge otowick onto which eardops containing an antiobiotic and steroid mixture are applied. Splinting will be necessary when there is EAM oedema preventing an adequate view of the tympanic membrane on otoscopy implying that ear drops will not reach the deeper recesses of the ear canal. The dressing should be changed at least every 48 hours until the canal swelling has settled sufficiently to allow any applied drops to reach the anteroinferior recess directly.

3. The ears should be kept scrupulously dry until resolution. Swimming is inadvisable and precautions taken when bathing to prevent water entering the ear canal.

In most reactive conditions the above regime is also recommended in order to prevent secondary infection of a raw ear canal surface.

Follow-up and aftercare

Treatment should continue for at least one week after resolution because of the tendency to recurrence particularly in otomycosis (fungal infection of the ear). Itchy reactive conditions may benefit from a course of Beclomethasone ear drops and an 8% solution of Aluminium Acetate or Acetic Acid ear spray is recommended in patients with chronic otitis externa after the acute infection has been eradicated.

NECROTISING OTITIS EXTERNA

This is an otitis externa which progresses to an osteomyelitis initially of the tympanic plate which is across the floor of the bony ear canal. This may spread to involve the skull base. It is most common after middle age, in diabetics and is usually caused by P. aeruginosa. The overwhelming symptom is a constant deep otalgia and it may cause 7-12th cranial nerve palsies, meningitis, sigmoid sinus thrombosis, brain abscess and death.

The condition should be suspected in a patient with granulation tissue deep in the external meatus which does not settle with the usual treatment. The diagnosis is often not considered until a cranial nerve palsy has developed. When such a patient develops a facial nerve palsy the differential diagnosis is between Acute Suppurative Otitis media(almost always secondary to a dehiscent horizontal portion of the facial nerve), Chronic Suppurative Otitis Media and Necrotising Otitis Externa and carcinoma. Histological and microbiological examination of the granulation tissue and a high definition CT scan of the temporal bone are required to make the diagnosis.

Treatment

Intravenous antibiotics as determined by the culture and sensitivity results are used. The dose and duration of treatment is decided by monitoring clinical response but often therapy has to be continued for months. Even with aggressive treatment there is still a significant mortality. Opiate analgesia may be required to control the deep otalgia.

MIDDLE EAR CONDITIONS AND OPERATIONS ENCOUNTERED

CHOLESTEATOMA

Cholesteatoma describes a collection of skin (keratinising squamous epithelium) within the middle ear. It develops from a retraction pocket when the upper part of the drum has been sucked inwards due to negative pressure in the middle ear. As it enlarges the cholesteatoma erodes the structures it encounters, especially bone. This damages the ossicles as well as exposing the inner ear, the facial nerve and the meninges of the brain. The contents of the cholesteatoma have no blood supply and become easily infected by any bacteria which happen to be around. Infection spreads to the various exposed structures. When the cholesteatoma becomes infected foul-smelling pus will be discharged.

The patient complains of deafness and/or foul-smelling discharge. There may be earache. On examination an attic or marginal perforation is found. CT scanning of the temporal bone shows a cavity where the affected mastoid bone has been eroded, usually a sclerotic (small mastoid air cells) mastoid is found.

Treatment is usually surgical and aims to make the ear safe. Conservative treatment such as repeated micro-suction can be used in the elderly and infirm or as a temporising means prior to surgery.

MASTOIDECTOMY

In this operation the diseased and infected tissues are removed leaving a cavity. In a modified radical mastoidectomy there is preservation of as much of the undiseased middle ear contents as is possible. The cavity may be repaired or obliterated and the ossicles replaced either at the time of the mastoidectomy or at a second sitting. There may be a cavity that needs cleaning for the rest of the patients' life. Although the mastoidectomy will usually give the patient a safe ear this may be at the price of a hearing loss.

TYMPANOPLASTY

The operation of tympanoplasty is designed to reconstruct the middle ear and so improve hearing. It must be carried out on a safe ear, preferably a dry one. It involves the repair to the drum perforation and the reconstruction of the defects in the ossicular chain. Fascia from the temporalis muscle which is readily accessible above the pinna is used for the graft to repair the drum. A bed is first prepared for the fascia by de-epithelialisation of the perforations edges, so ensuring skin cannot grow into the middle ear. Some types of tympanoplasty will include ossicular reconstruction as well as drum repair.

PERFORATIONS

Characterised as either central or marginal.

Central Perforation – Need not be in the centre of thetympanic membrane. It is a perforation that has a rim (however narrow) of normal drum between the edge of the perforation and the bony annulus.

Marginal – No drum between it and bony annulus – extends to the bony margin. The distinction between the two types of perforation is important because marginal perforations are more likely to produce cholesteatomas, especially posterior marginal perforations.

TWO TYPES OF PERFORATION

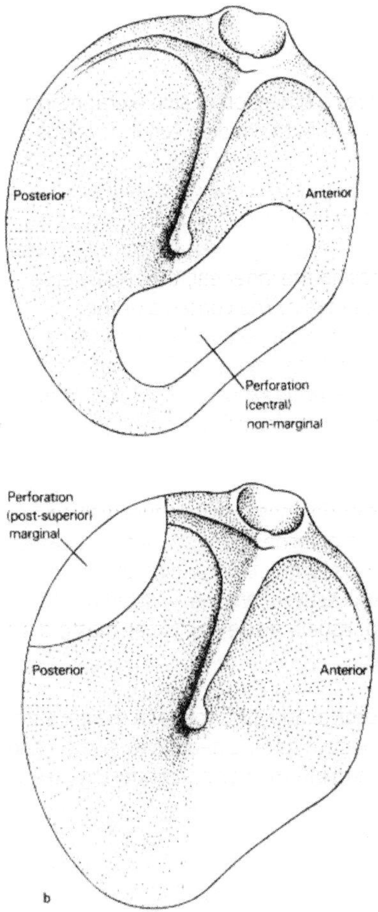

THE PATIENT WITH OTORRHOEA

Definition

Otorrhoea is the discharge of material from the ear. It is both a symptom and a sign but It is not a diagnosis.

Causes

Otitis externa and suppurative otitis media are the commonest diseases causing this problem. Other causes include: wax, debris, blood (acute otitis media, trauma, neoplasm), and CSF (usually following a fracture).

Clinical features

The character of the discharge depends on (and therefore gives clues to) its source.

1. **External ear**. There are no mucinous glands in the external canal. Acute inflammatory conditions of the external canal therefore tend to produce a watery, serous exudates or transudate. In addition, they tend to provoke a hyperkeratosis, more skin formation. This combination generally leads to soggy white debris collecting in the canal and a thin white watery discharge from the ear. The cardinal symptom of otitis externa is itchiness, in addition to the discharge, pain and tenderness. The external canal may also be the subject of trauma, which may lead to bleeding from the ear.

2. **Middle ear**. The middle ear cleft is well endowed with mucous glands. Thus, if there is a mucoid component to the discharge it usually arises from the middle ear via a perforation of the tympanic membrane. Trapped keratin is offensive; if a cholesteatoma becomes infected the discharge tends to be particularly unpleasant and once smelt is never forgotten. A serosanguinous discharge is common with chronic otitis media when the middle ear mucosa has become granular and polypoid; there is glandular hyperplasia and there may be blood as the mucosa bleeds easily. Blood stained discharge is also a feature of carcinoma of the middle ear. Chronic otitis media is not typically characterized by pain, so in patients where chronic otorrhoea becomes painful and fails to respond to the usual conservative measures, it is wise to consider a carcinoma.

3. **Cerebrospinal fluid**. CSF rarely discharges from the ears spontaneously but may do so following skull base surgery or more commonly trauma, when it will develop in about 5% of cases. In both cases the fluid may initially be mixed with blood and may be recognized by the halo sign in which there is a clear ring of moisture surrounding the blood after absorption on to blotting paper or the patients pillow. This is due to the faster diffusion of the less viscous CSF. Differentiation of CSF from thin serous discharge from a middle ear cavity may be more difficult but can be done by confirming the presence of, ß2-transferrin in CSF. If the tympanic membrane is intact CSF may still leak from the ear should there be a fracture in the roof of the ear canal. Otherwise it will pass down the Eustachian tube and become evident as rhinorrhoea or post-nasal drip.

Management

Optimum management depends on making an accurate diagnosis. Although the history will give many clues, the diagnosis is usually not made until the tympanic membrane has been visualized. This may not be possible at the initial consultation owing to swelling and debris in the external auditory meatus. A swab should be taken for culture and sensitivity (bacteria/fungi). This is especially important in patients who have already been on treatments which have not worked. Any granulation type tissue removed should be sent for histology. The mainstay of therapy is aural toilet, ideally by microsuction clearance. This enables a thorough assessment, diagnosis of cause, and allows better penetration of any topical treatments.

Treatment will often commence on the basis of a best guess diagnosis. This will invariably require attention to the primary or secondary otitis externa by thorough aural toilet and possibly the insertion of a wick. At the time of definitive diagnosis more appropriate treatment can be continued. Treatment of the otitis externa will be sufficient if this is the diagnosis. Middle ear disease will demand treatment on its own merits.

Patients with CSF otorrhoea are at risk of meningitis. Post traumatic leaks usually resolve spontaneously within a short period but surgical repair will be required if they continue.

WAX REMOVAL; EVIDENCE BASED GUIDELINES

Rationale

Wax removal is a common clinical procedure in primary health care and within ear, nose and throat departments. Literature suggests that between 25,000 and 40,000 patients ears are syringed each week in the United Kingdon.(Grossan, 1998; Memel, Langley, Watkins et al, 2002). A paper published in 1990 (Sharp et al) found that on average, a general practitioner sees nine patients a month requiring ear syringing or wax removal. No previous evidence based guidelines exist for the management of a patient with wax problems.

Guideline users should be aware that recommendations might not be appropriate for use in all circumstances.

Taking the general heading into account of WAX REMOVAL and the fact that the guidelines have to have an impact on the quality of care and patient practices there was a need to identify and review published literature so that the recommendations could be based on the evidence available.

THE SEARCH STRATEGY

The search strategy attempted to locate systematic reviews, meta-analysis, randomised trials and studies using a combination of key words. Also, contact was made with other specialists including the medical devices agency for relevant safety notices and the Medical Defence Union and Medical Protection Society, as to litigation concerns. Searches were linked to English language citations only and electronic searches of the following databases were performed:

- PUB – MED
- CINAHL
- COCHRANE TRIALS REGISTER

All databases were searched from 1966 to the present day.

Ear Syringing	Wax
Aural care/toilet	Ear wax
Ear canal	Ear meatus
External auditory canal	Propulse
Cerumen	Otitis externa
Ear drops	Wax softners
Cerumenolytics	Wax removal

Above is a list of key words used.

The whole search revealed 938 papers from the three databases. The database literature was sifted for relevance to the clinical area of the guideline – the key word wax revealed 48 results on the CINAHL database but entries included wax baths and Rheumatology treatments. Titles concerned with non-relevant clinical areas were removed. The sifting process also included removing duplicate articles found on one or more of the databases or the articles that appeared under more than one key word i.e. wax and aural care.

We did not attempt to use unpublished reports or abstracts. After sifting the literature and rejecting abstracts we were left with 43 papers relevant to the clinical problem. The library was contacted for these papers.

GRADING

Papers are graded by the strength of their evidence (see appendix 1a). It revealed 16 papers that would be of value in providing guidelines.

One paper at level one
One paper at level two
One paper at level three
Two papers providing guidelines prodigy and clinical evidence
The remaining eleven papers contained only level five plus evidence.

This highlighted the distinct lack of evidence and good research in this area.

Most of the papers were written from experience and lacked any evidence to support their claims.

The draft guidelines on wax removal were written, giving consideration as to the strength of the recommendation (see below)

The strength of evidence provided in these guidelines was interpreted in the light of the clinical arena. It was accepted that due to the limited number of papers relating to the clinical problem of wax removal that a guideline may not receive a high recommendation.

WAX REMOVAL – IS IT NECESSARY?

Wax is a normal physiologicall substance and should only be removed if it is causing the patient symptoms, (Level A recommendation) or if it prevents inspection of the tympanic membrane, (Level D recommendation)

Rationale

Wax removal has been shown to improve hearing in those patients with impacted wax. Memel et al (2002) demonstrated a mean improvement in hearing of 6.9 decibels after wax removal. A postal survey by Sharp et al (1990) concluded that removal of wax improved patients hearing by a mean of 5.45 decibels. Both indicate a clinically significant improvement in hearing as a result of wax removal.

Patients seek wax removal for a range of symptoms including hearing problems, blocked ears, noises in the ears, itchy ears, dizziness and ear pain. (Sharp et al, 1990, Browning, 2001, Memel et al, 2002. These symptoms are not easy to quantify and objectively assess. One randomised controlled trial (Memel et al 2002) looked at patients' subjective benefits to wax removal

Patients subjective reports as to their change in symptoms included –

1. Difficulty hearing on the phone
   75% experienced improvement
2. Pain
   70% experienced improvement
3. Blocked ears
   62% experienced improvement
4. Difficulty hearing one to one
   61% experienced improvement
5. Difficulty hearing in a group
   55% experienced improvement
6. Noises
   49% experienced improvement
7. Dizziness
   48% experienced improvement
8. Itchy ears
   39% experienced improvement

Cited in Memel et alC 2002

Objective measurements are based on an evidence level one paper and a postal survey; these two papers provided consistent evidence that wax removal improved hearing. Subjective reports as to improvement in hearing and blocked ears correlated well with objective measurements.

WAX SOFTNERS – WHICH CERUMINOLYTIC?

A Ceruminolytic should be advised if the wax is hard and impacted. Sodium bicarbonate being the cerumonolytic of choice in the acute phase, optimum time for use is 5 days. Olive oil, being the lubricant of choice, for chronic problems. (Level D recommendation)

Rationale

The literature search revealed no objective, unbiased, randomised controlled trials as to the best wax softener. Browning (2001) defines this lack of evidence: Use of a wax softener versus no treatment reduced risk of impaction if used for five days. A ceruminolytic should soften, loosen, liquefy and disintegrate wax. The survey conducted by Sharp (1990) indicated that the most commonly advised ceruminolytic was olive oil.

Hawke (2002) provided in-vitro evidence that the use of sodium bicarbonate and water are better than oil. He found that the chemical composition of wax responded better to aqueous solutions such as water and sodium bicarbonate as they provided better breakdown of the wax. Oil based solutions only lubricated the wax. In Vitro studies proved that olive oil appeared to be totally ineffective in dispersing earwax, water was more effective. Eeekhof, et al (2001) in a prospective randomised trial concluded water used for 15 minutes prior to syringing in patients with persistent wax, worked well in daily practice with real patients.

Of the propriety brands, Sharp et al (1990) found that Cerumol was the drug of choice given by doctors. However a large multi-centre trial found Exterol to be significantly more effective and Cerumol (Fahmy, 1982). Studies have revealed sodium bicarbonate more effective than oil, if instilled correctly. The BNF (2002) states that both preparations are equally safe and inexpensive. The joint Formulary Committee feels proprietary brands are less suitable for prescribing and should not be the first drug of choice (BNF 2002), as they may cause irritation and inflammation to the external ear canal. There was no level 1 evidence that wax softeners work better than placebo. The consensus is that they do.

ASSESSMENT OF SUITABILITY FOR EAR SYRINGING

A full Otological history and examination should be undertaken prior to syringing the ear.

CHECK FOR CONTRAINDICATIONS TO MINIMISE COMPLICATIONS

- Patient history as to previous and current ear problems and conditions – read patient notes and ask patient
- End-aural and post auricular examination for signs of an incision, which would indicate previous surgery; skin problems indicating otitis externa, severe pain on manipulation of pinna
- Otoscopy to assess wax and any stenosis of the ear canal, or mucopurulent discharge in ear canal, which usually signifies middle ear disease
- Document findings in a structured format
- If in doubt about suitability – DO NOT SYRINGE
- (Level D recommendation)

Rationale

It has been acknowledged in the literature that complications do arise from ear syringing (Sharp et al, 1990; Price, 1997; Blake et al, 1998; Grossan 1996). However, the incidence is unknown. Evidence found due to litigation claims points to the need for accurate otological assessment. Practitioners should know the contra-indications to ear syringing to decrease complications.

Blake et al (1998) when dealing with litigation claims during the period 1992-1993 discussed that out of 47 accepted ear syringing claims, 17 ears were syringed with the patients having a clear otological history, others had persistent otitis externa. It was concluded in general that the practice documentation was inadequate and often markedly different from the claimants' version. This is confirmed by Price (1997), who says that the main causes for complications that the Medical Defence Union found were failure to take a full history or examine the ear, so the contraindications to syringing were not found. 69% of practitioners who were involved in litigation were found to have poor record keeping and history taking was not documented. Practice falls short of what is ideal. Complications found in Sharpe's survey (1990) indicated that 38% of the GP's had encountered complications, however, included in the complications was a failure to remove wax. The next highest complication was a perforated tympanic membrane (Sharpe et al, 1990). The evidence provided by Price (1997) that the most common adverse outcome was a perforated tympanic membrane – happened in 35% of the claims.

Evidence provided in a level 2 study by Vibeke et al (1995) who performed in vitro syringing showed the pressure developed in the external auditory meatus was insufficient to rupture a NORMAL tympanic membrane. They concluded if a perforation arose it was due to the fact that the tympanic membrane was not normal prior to the procedure. Weakening occurs as a consequence of a healed perforation, recurrent infections, otitis media with effusion; grommets may extrude leaving a thinner tympanic membrane segment. Unhealed perforations are a marked contra-indication. (Blake et al 1998) Evidence strongly points to the fact that complications are avoided by obtaining a full otological history and examining the ear for prior pathology (Grossan, 1998). Collection of data in a structured format will enable consideration of clinical factors that may impact on need to syringe ears. If the patient gives a poor history and the tympanic membrane cannot be examined due to wax impaction, and if there is no previous documented visual examination of the eardrum available – do not syringe the ear.

Contraindications

History of perforated ear drum
Previous or pending ear surgery
Previous or current history of ear disease
Otitis externa
Previous injury or a stated aversion to ear syringing
Only hearing ear
Stenosed ear canals – may be a result of infections or bony exostosis
Foreign bodies – sharp or hygroscopic in nature
Known inner ear disturbance causing severe vertigo

SYRINGING – METAL OR ELECTRIC?

There is no evidence that electric is better or worse than the metal syringe.

The most important factor when using either syringe is that the person using it is trained and experienced to operate it.

Other factors include:

- That the syringing equipment is properly maintained
- Check that the syringe is assembled correctly, prior to use, ensuring the nozzle is firmly attached
- Verbal consent is obtained
- Correct technique is used
- Procedure is stopped if patient experiences any problems
- Check ears after syringing to see if wax is removed, and that no complications have arisen
- Dry any excess water from the ear
- Document procedure, which syringe used, attempts and any adverse problems during procedure

(Level D recommendation)

Rationale

No evidence was found that the metal is better or worse than the electric ear syringe. The randomised trial looking at the effectiveness of ear syringing in general practice used both the metal and electric syringe with no detrimental effects noted with either. (Memel et al 2002). In 1998 a study by Kent found that nurses were divided in their use of ear syringing equipment, they made their choice on the confidence they had in using the syringe and the results obtained and thus their choice was not based on research. No papers were found relating to metal ear syringe versus electric ear syringe. Vibeke et al (1995) provided good evidence that normal pressure produced by the metal ear syringe is insufficient to rupture a healthy eardrum. They concluded that they could confirm that ear syringing in general was a safe practice.

Blake et al (1998) in their litigation claims found that the evidence points to that the metal syringe will not perforate a healthy eardrum if used properly.

The main evidence found points to poor maintenance and assembly of equipment prior to syringing. A medical devices agency safety notice (SN 9807) issued in February 1998 in regards to the 'Propulse' suggested that the low and top end stops are checked before every use, as excessive force on the output control can break the end stop and cause damage in the ear. No notices have been declared on the updated model the Propulse II. A report by Dinsdale (1991) discusses a patient receiving injuries, in the external ear canal with a dental tip from an electric syringe. Price (1997) quotes one incidence of negligence due to poor assembly of equipment.

"Nozzle of a metal syringe came adrift during ear syringing causing a perforation". The metal syringe must be lubricated properly and nozzle firmly attached prior to each syringing. The Propulse II in its manufacturers guidelines indicates the need to attach a jet tip, also, it has available for use a disposable angled jet tip, for one use only, again care in assembly is required.

Bapat, (2001) provide further evidence that complications arise despite no contraindications but due to faulty technique they report on a case of a patient suffering audio-vestibular damage due to the nozzle of a syringe being inserted too far down the external auditory canal and traumatising the ossicles and fracturing the stapes bone. Blake et al (1995) support this when discussing the technique of syringing that the nozzle should not be inserted too deep into the canal and that the pinna should be pulled up and back and the syringe directed along the postero-superior canal wall, so the syringe is not pointed directly at the tympanic membrane. Again advocating the need for thorough training programmes. The literature suggests that syringing may precipitate an infection, so the ear should be dried after syringing to remove residual water. The equipment should be decontaminated appropriately as per manufacturers' instructions. Manual ear syringing equipment should not be stored wet. Propulse manufacturers' instructions stress that water at the end of the day should be discarded as to be left could build up bacteria, including pseudomonas, a common reason for patients requiring treatment for otitis externa, again no studies were available to provide evidence as to the incidence of this.

Whilst there is no evidence that wax syringing in an otherwise normal ear causes deafness there are occasional circumstantial treatment case reports of this. It is therefore prudent to warn the patient that unforeseen problems can occur with any procedure and these could include deafness, dizziness, tinnitus, perforation and infection but that these are very rare.

SUMMARY

Wax should be removed if this is causing the patient symptoms. These symptoms may include difficulty hearing, pain blocked ears, noises, dizziness and itchy ears. Wax softeners can be used for a period of five days, Sodium bicarbonate being the cerumenolytic of choice in the acute phase and olive oil being the lubricant of choice for chronic problems, or if any otitis externa has occurred.

When assessing the suitability for ear syringing and being aware of the contra-indications, ear syringing can be done either with the electric or hand syringe and excess water should be dried away. Documentation is mandatory.

Clinical Guidelines for Wax removal on Manual Removal of Wax

Manual removal is appropriate for patients with contra-indications to syringing. There is no evidence to demonstrate this is better or worse than syringing in normal patients but in patients with contra-indications to syringing it is the only option available. This is where aural care clinics come in.

Clinical Guidance – Wax Removal

Categories of Evidence

I Evidence from meta analysis of randomised controlled trials or form at least one randomised controlled trial

II Evidence from at least one controlled study without randomisation or at least one other type of quasi-experimental study

III Evidence from non-experimental descriptive studies, such as comparative studies, correlation studies and case control studies.

IV Evidence from expert committee reports or opinions and/or clinical experience of respected authorities.

Strength of Recommendations

A: Directly based on category I evidence
B: Directly based on category II evidence or extrapolated recommendation from category I evidence
C: Directly based on category III evidence or extrapolated recommendation from category I or II evidence
D: Directly based on category IV evidence or extrapolated recommendation from category I, II or III evidence

PHOTOGRAPHS

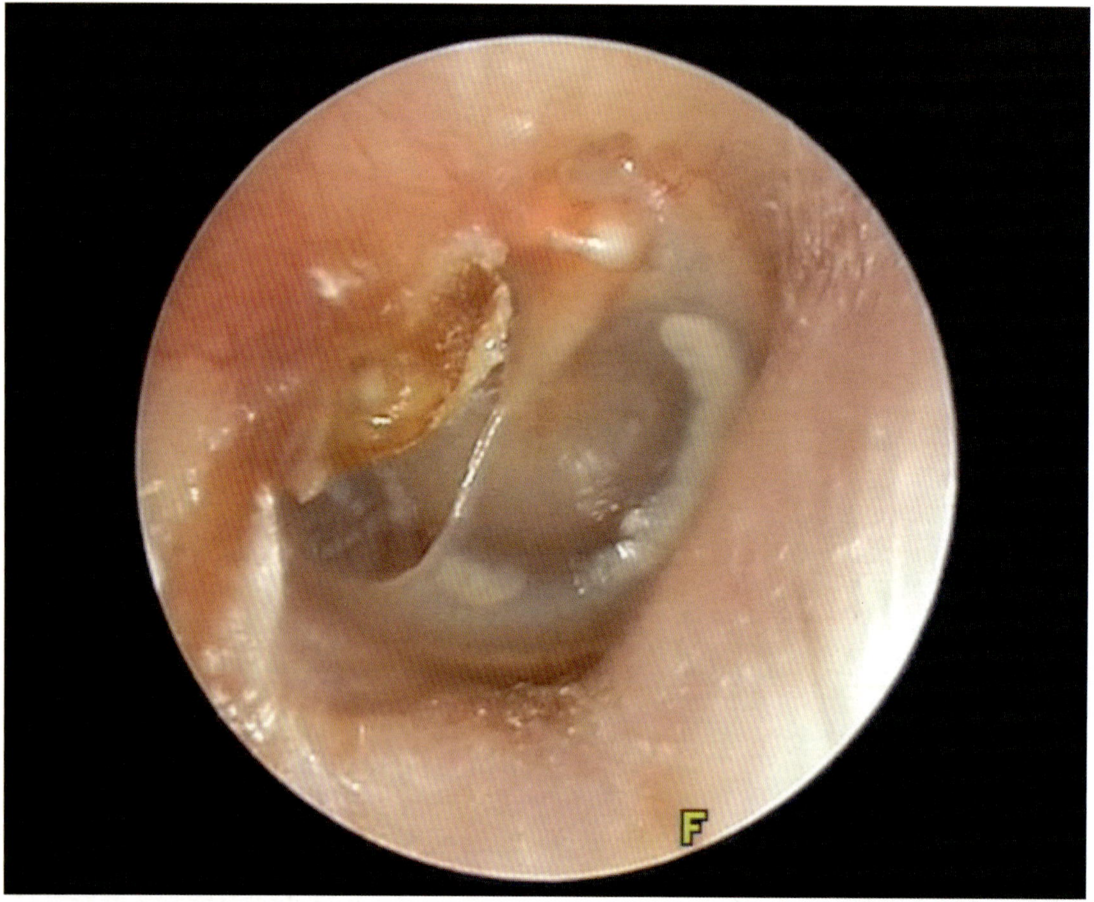

Keratin/wax hiding small cholesteatoma in right ear

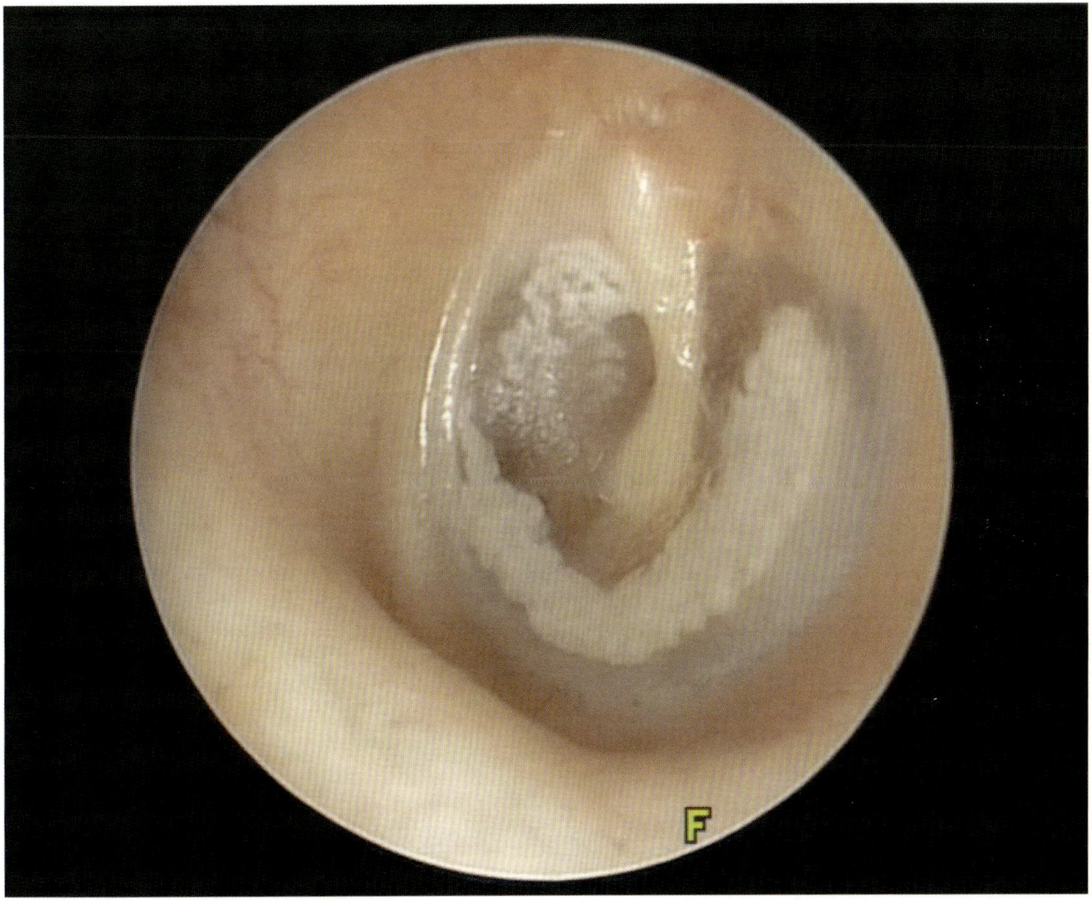

Horseshoe shaped tympanosclerosis in left ear.

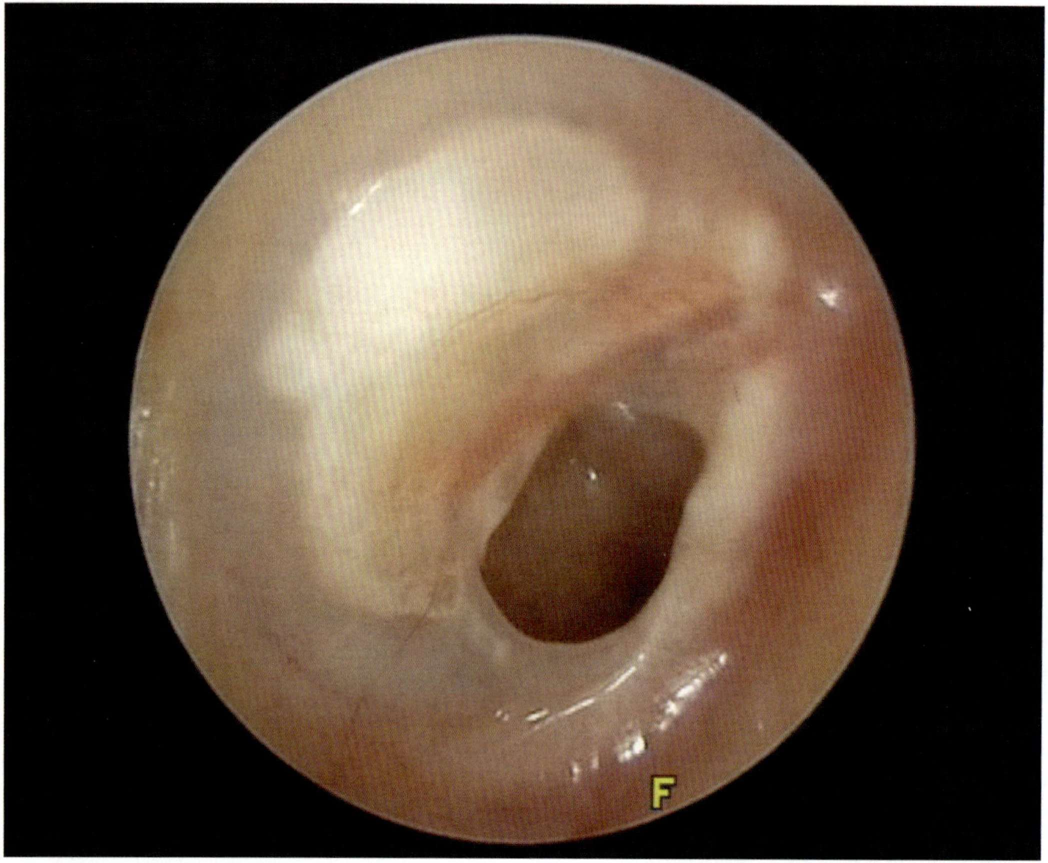

Anterior perforation in right ear with tympanosclerosis affecting the posterior part of the ear drum.

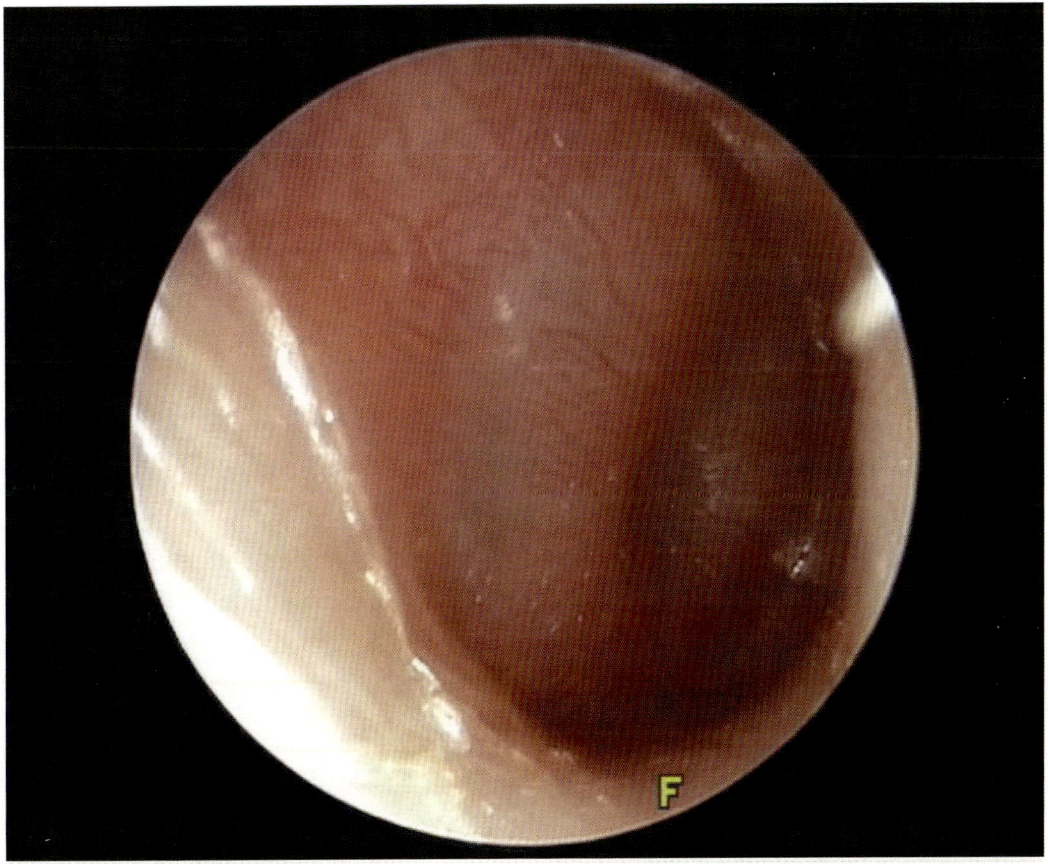

Bulging right ear drum with glue ear, note seashore effect of the posterior part of the ear canal.

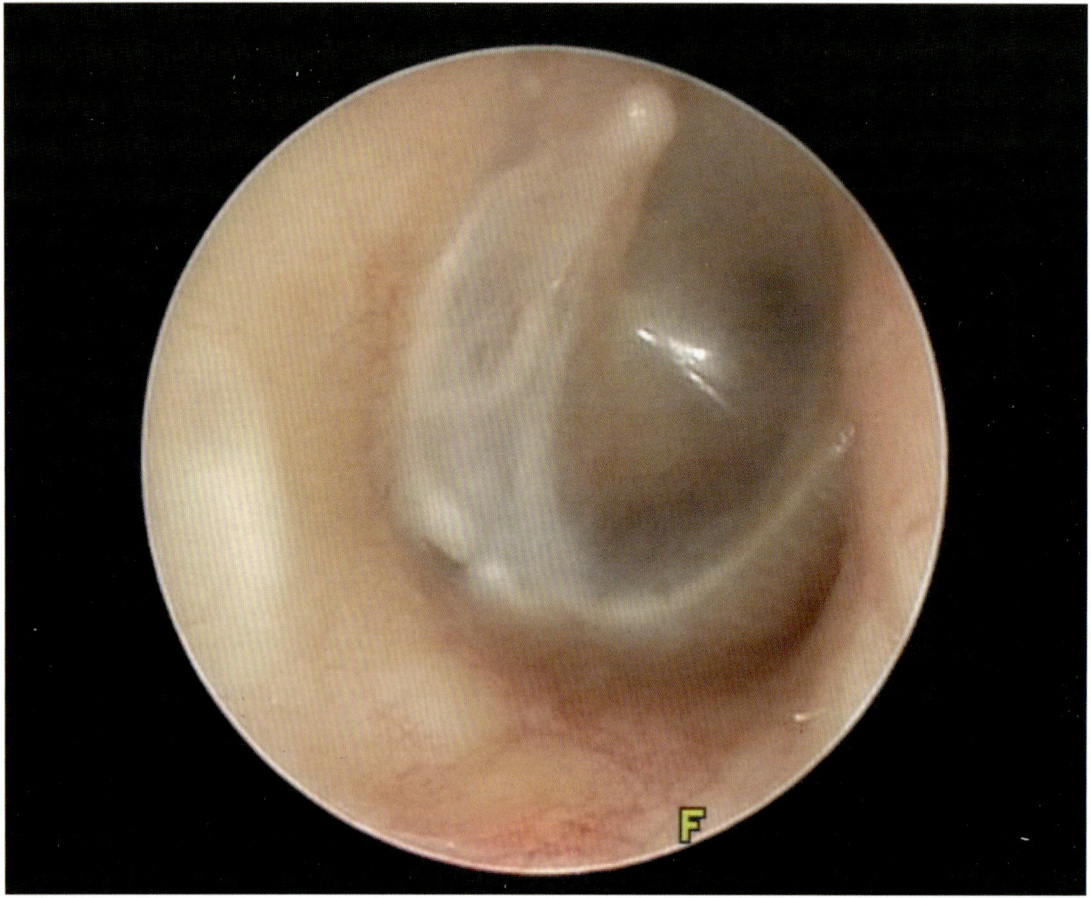

Annular ligament is disrupted, this patient has had stapes surgery 20 years ago.

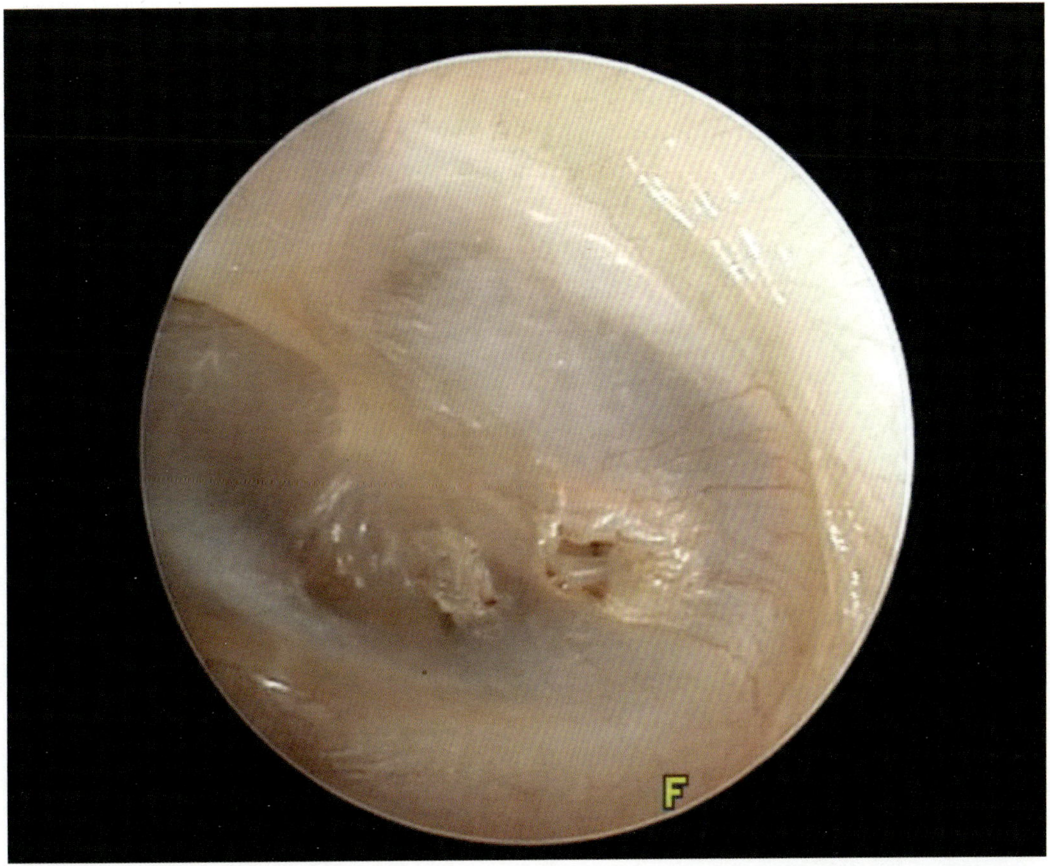

Traumatic perforation two weeks ago following football being kicked against ear, keratin is building up around the hole as it spontaneously heals.

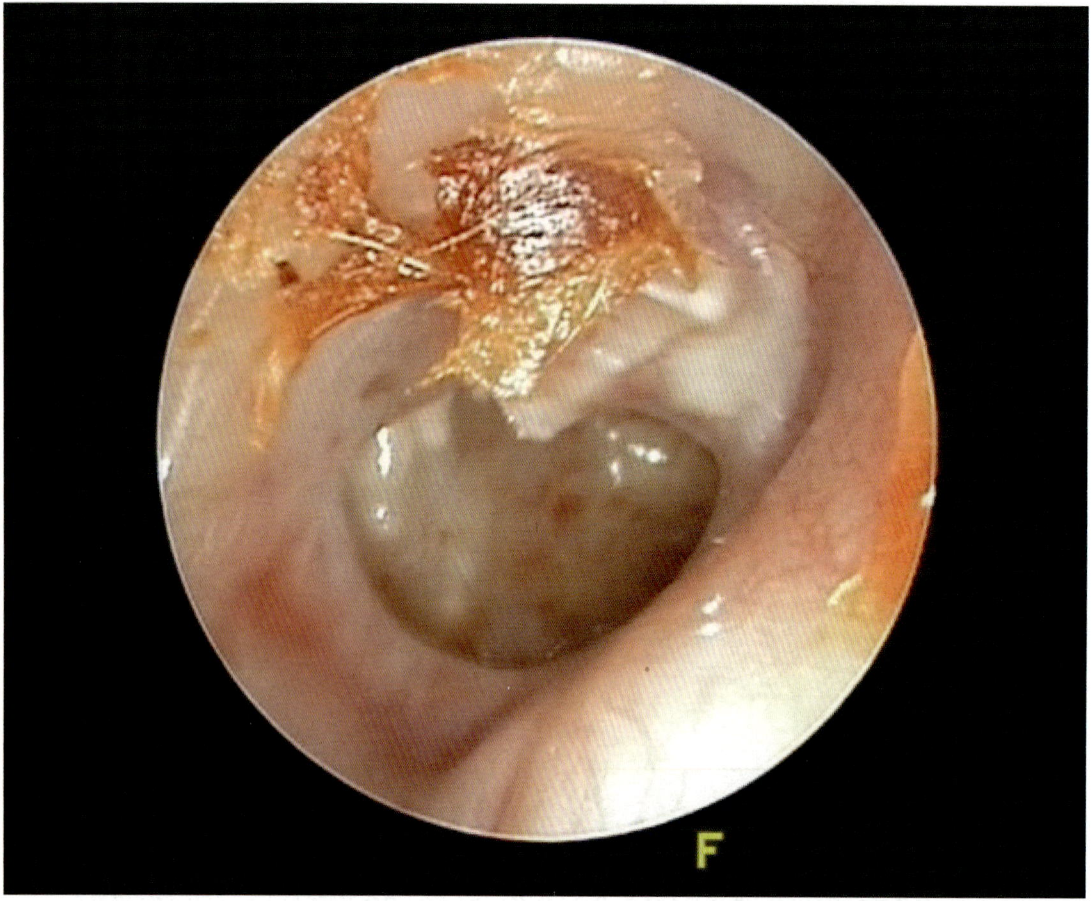

Right ear drum with large perforation still with wax superiorly.

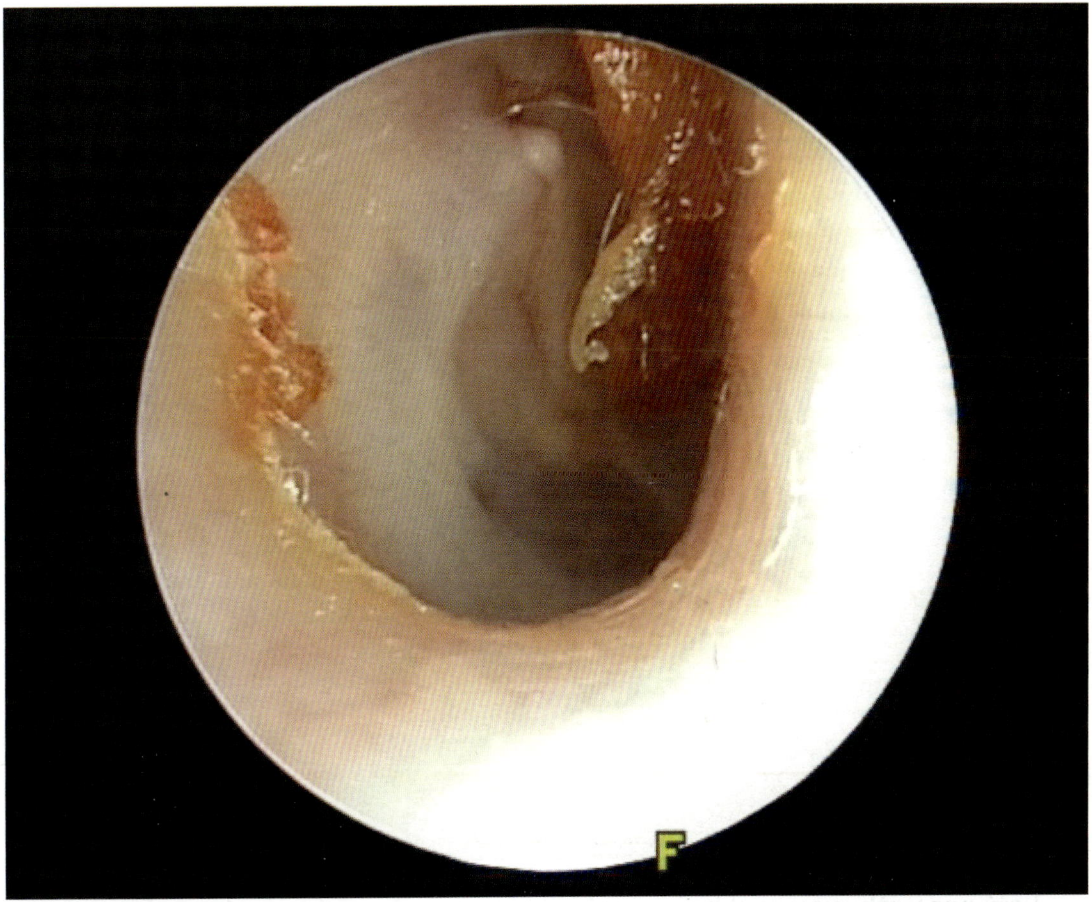

Wax in anterior recess, patient previously had myringoplasty.

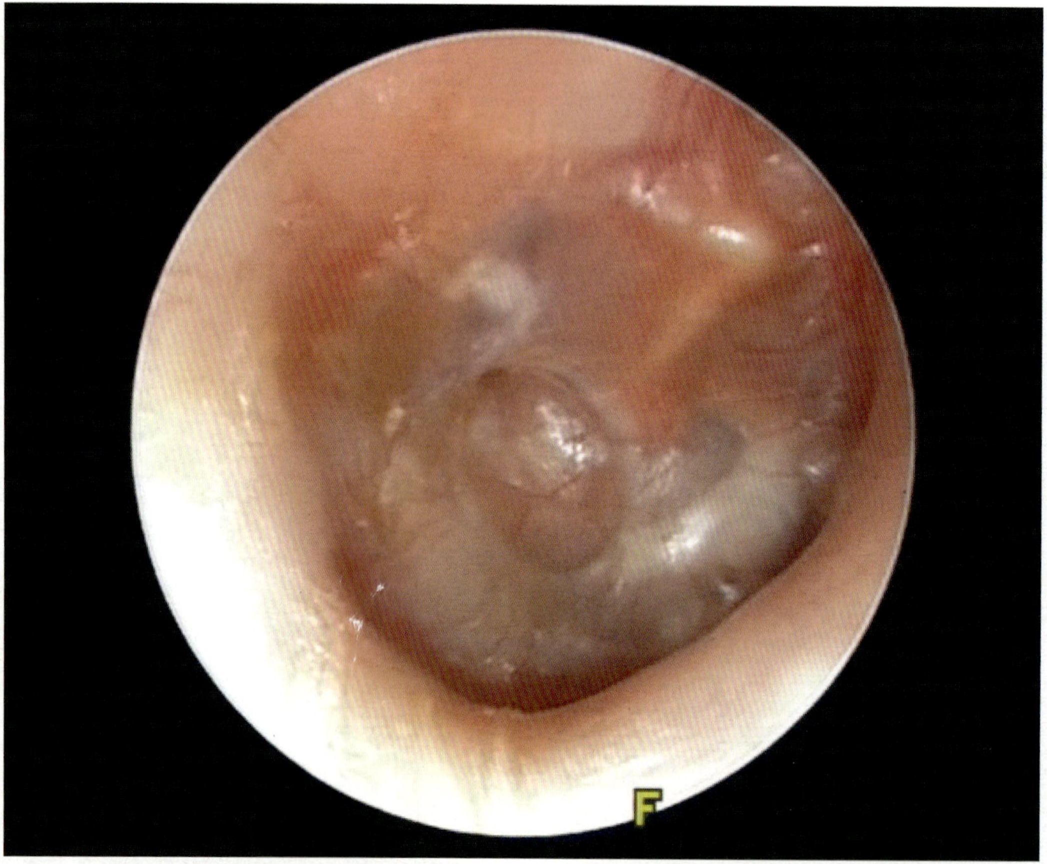

Patient with previous tympanoplasty for cholesteatoma has scarred ear drum, no visible recurrence.

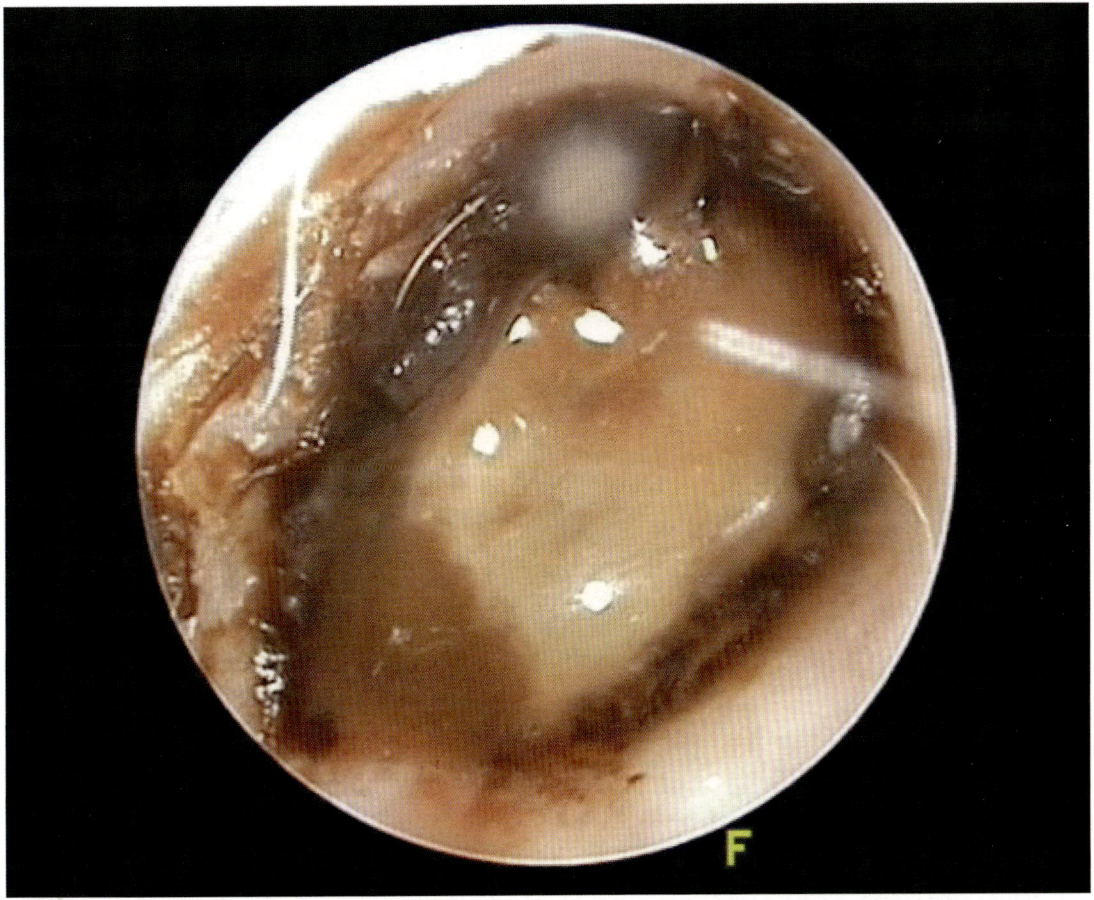

Wax and debris in chronically discharging ear.

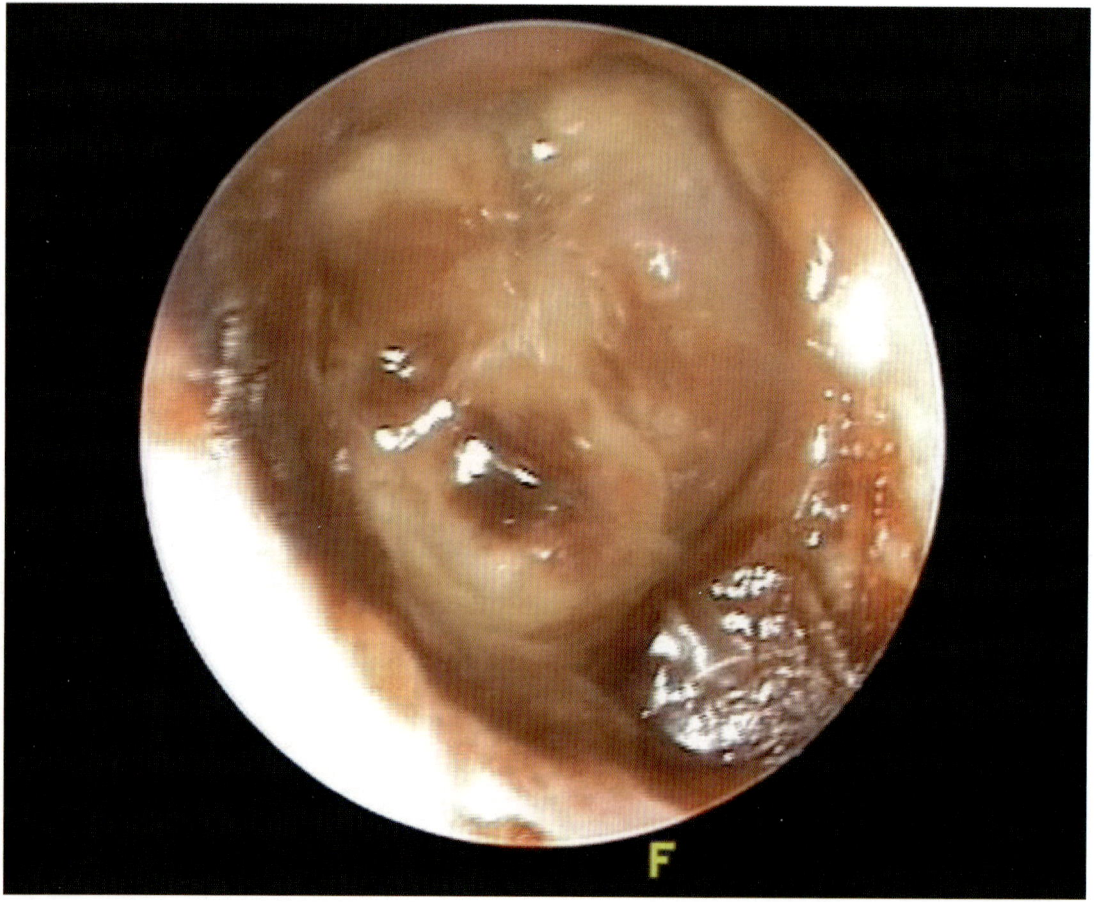

Infected wax and debris in mastoid cavity.

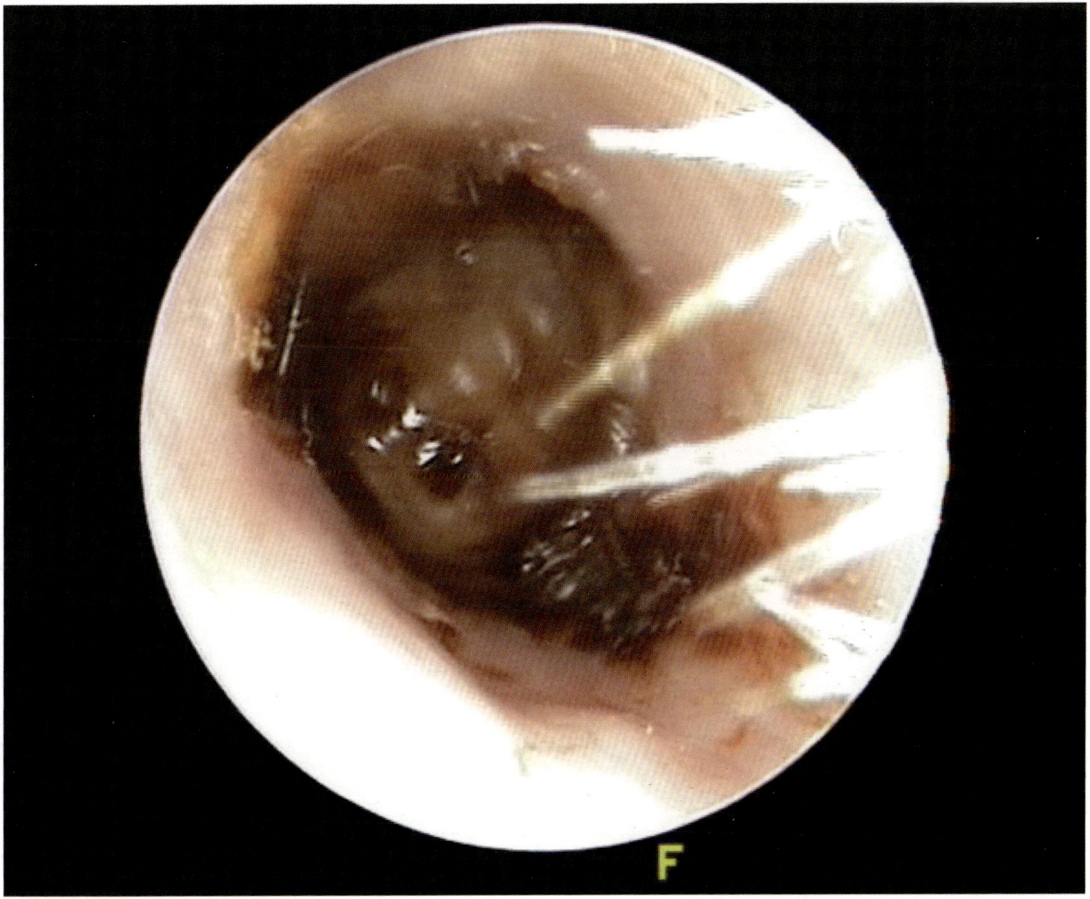

Debris in ear canal in chronic otitis externa.

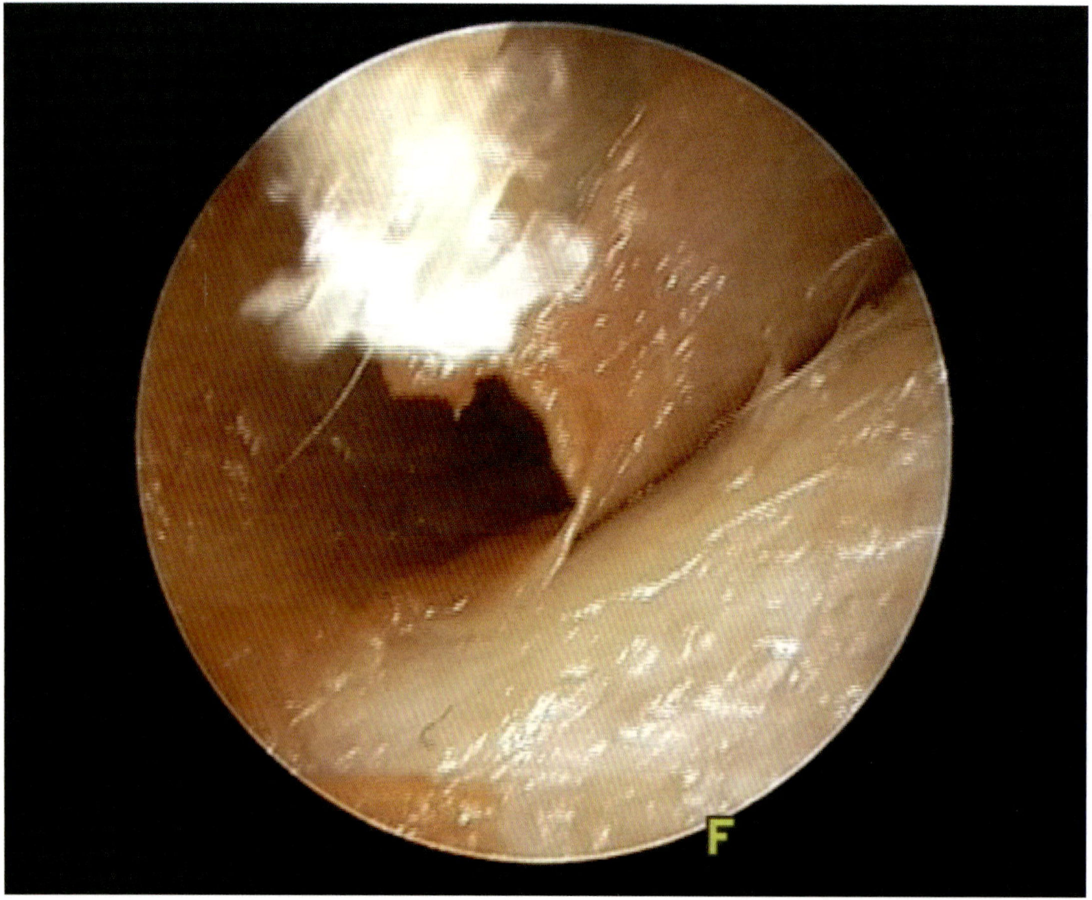

Wax and skin being lifted off ear canal in chronic otitis externa.

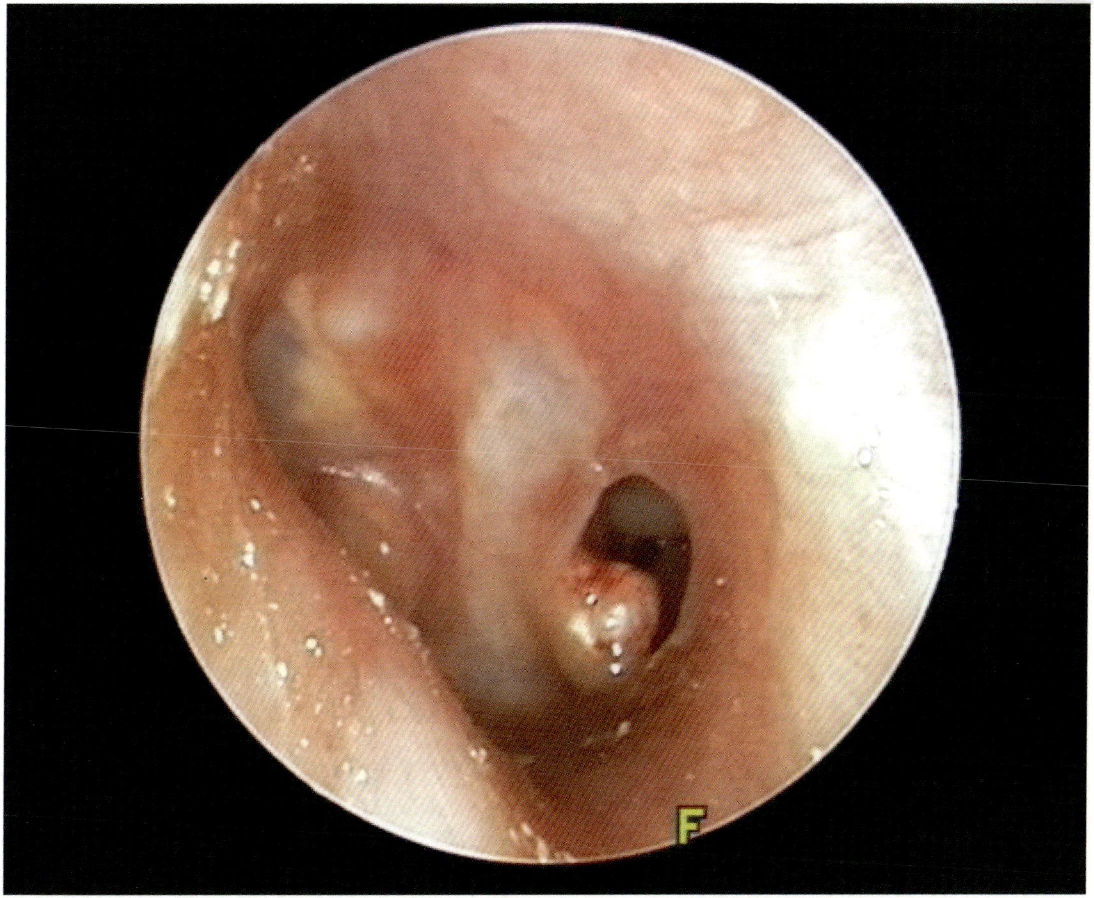

Hole in posterior part of ear drum after failed myringoplasty.

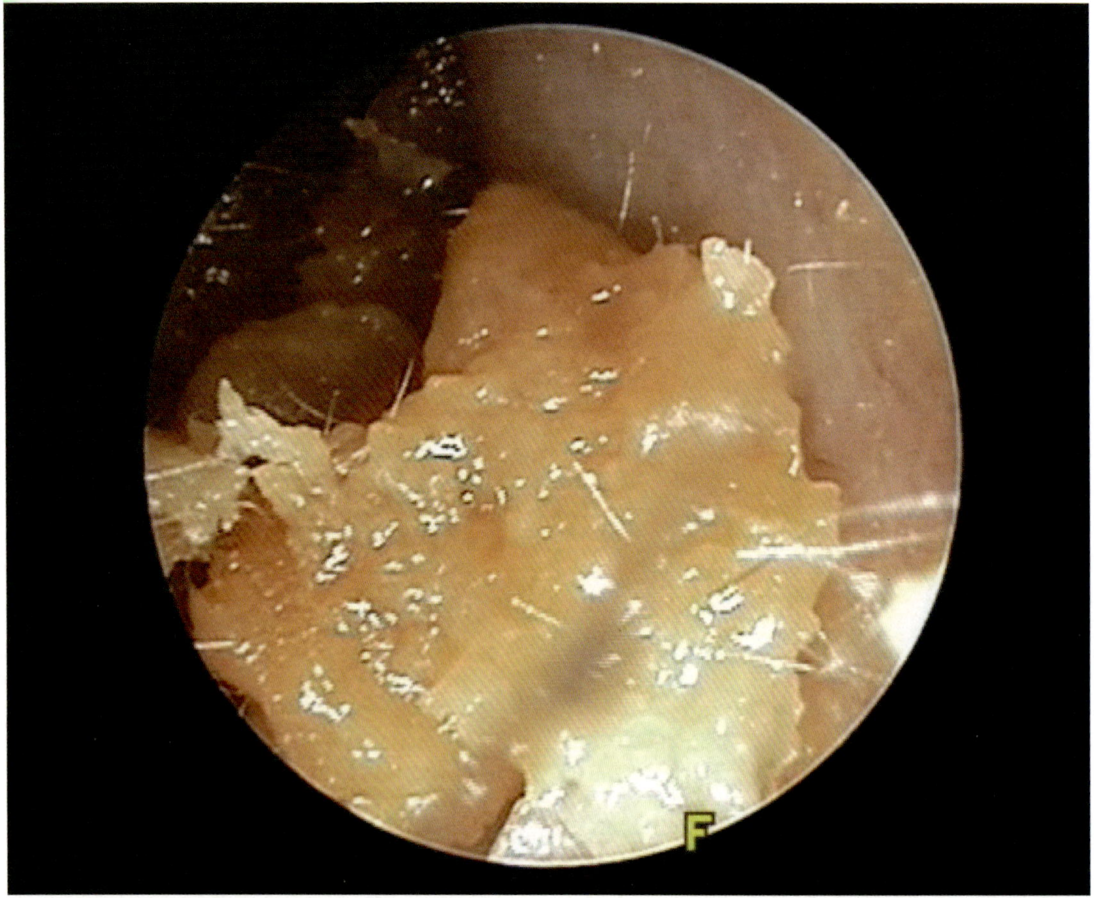

Wax containing hairs in ear canal.

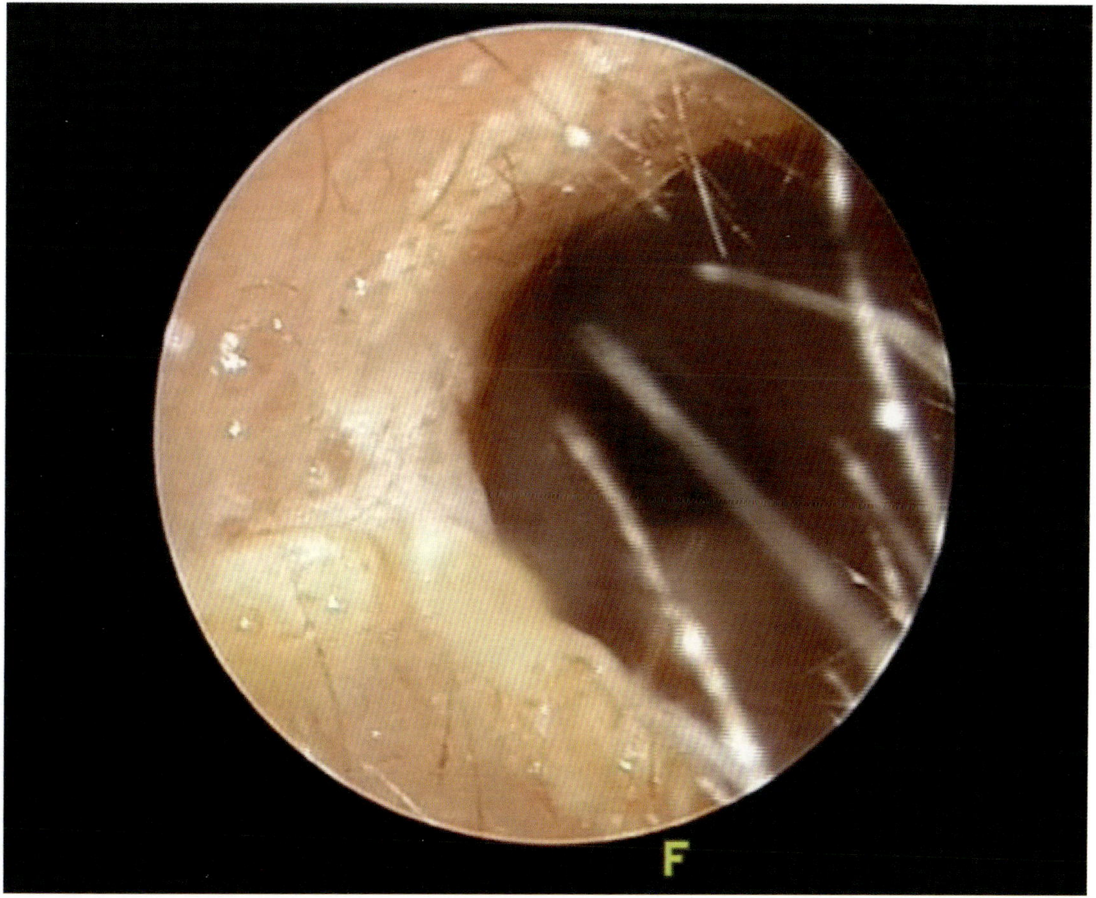

A very itchy ear.

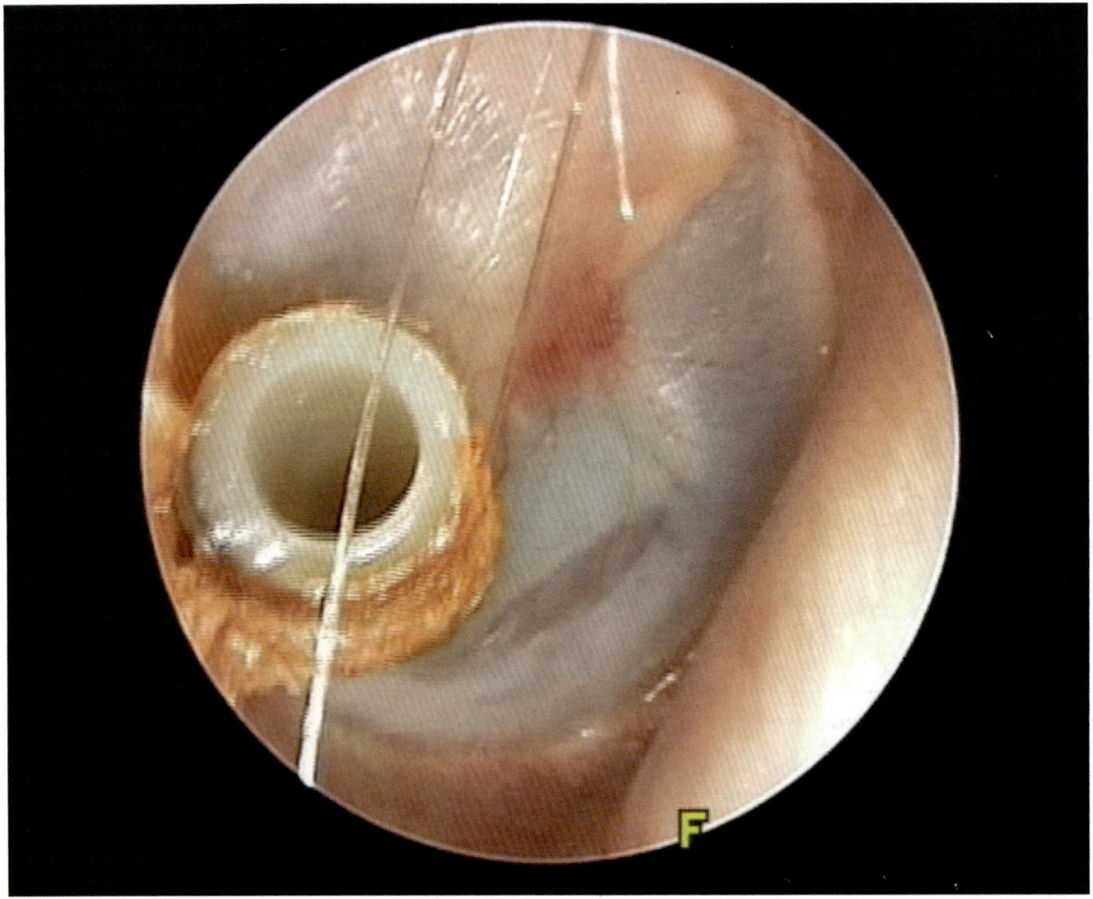

A tube grommet in posterior part of ear drum.

SOUTHPORT & ORMSKIRK NHS TRUST

New Patient Referral to Nurse Aural Care Clinic Assessment Record

Patients Details	Patients DetailsConsultant GP Referral Date Allergies Medications

Past Medical History

	Yes	No		Yes	No
Ear surgery/disease			Skin Problems		
Deafness			Nasal problems		
Dizziness			Any illnesses		
Tinnitus			Previous microsuction		

Details (if yes to any of the above)

Complaint/Condition (see referral letter)

Patients symptoms on assessment

Treatment

Follow up Appointment

Letter to GP

Signature...

Date ....

There is little evidence for the treatments once the patient has been sent to the aural care clinic. The following guidelines are merely the ones that were developed for the clinic in Southport and are reviewed and revised on a three yearly basis.

GENERAL GUIDELINES FOR AURAL MICROSUCTION

1. PRIOR TO TREATMENT BY A NURSE THE NURSE MUST DOCUMENT IN THE PATIENT'S NOTES

- verbal consent to treatment by the nurse
- history of past and present ear problems
- previous and current state of hearing
- any relevant past major medical problems
  (ie cardiac, chest, hiatus hernia, arthritis, allergies etc)
- current medication
- any contra-indications to microsuction:
  recent vertigo
  severe pre-existing pain
  bleeding
  possible/known damage to middle ear structures
  inability to lie down/lie still
  recent ear surgery

2. EXAMINATION OF THE EARS

- The nurse introduces herself as the person to be giving the treatment
- Patient is asked to lie down on the couch
- Wash hands
- The pinna and surrounding skin are assessed for any:
  swelling, inflammation, tenderness, ulceration, scarring, evidence of previous surgery/treatment
- **Document, sign and date findings**
- The microscope should be switched on taking care that the light is not directed at the patients face
- The speculum with the largest diameter that fits comfortably into the meatus should be used
- Examine the meatus for any:
  narrowing, nodules, redness, dryness, swelling, discharge, cysts, foreign objects, excessive wax,
  REMEMBER:
- The external ear does not have any mucous glands, therefore if there is a mucous discharge it must have originated from the middle ear and the patient must have a perforation with underlying middle ear infection or cholesteatoma – REFER after cleaning

- **Document, sign and date findings**
- Proceed according to the relevant guidelines, if unsure REFER to doctor's clinic

3. PATIENT EDUCATION

- Inform the patient how to care for ears
- Emphasise importance of and how to keep the ears dry
- Ensure the patient knows how to instil ear drops correctly
- Ensure the patient knows how to obtain further treatment
- Advise against the use of cotton buds
- Advise against unprescribed 'remedies'
- Discuss effects of lifestyle and stress on aural condition

4. DOCUMENTATION

RECORD ALL

- Observations made
- Treatments given
- Education/information given
- Treatment plan/discharge from clinic/SOS appointment
- **SIGN, DATE AND TIME ALL ENTRIES**

5. COMMUNICATION

- Send letter to GP outlining treatment given
- Arrange follow-up appointment
- Explain to patient how to get help in an emergency
- Give written instructions as appropriate

GUIDELINES FOR THE TREATMENT OF OTITIS EXTERNA

OTITIS EXTERNA

Otitis externa is an inflammation of the skin lining the external auditory canal (EAC), sometimes involving the pinna. It can be infective (bacterial, fungal or viral) or reactive (allergy or eczema). It can also occur as an acute episode or be a chronic condition. It is one of the most common ear complaints.

Predisposing factors include:
- trauma – cotton buds, ear syringing, hearing aids
- swimming – in susceptible individuals
- allergy – eczema, dermatitis, dandruff, psoriasis
- secondary – to middle ear disease

Symptoms:
- itchy, irritation – can be unbearable
- discharge
- deafness – if inflammation has occluded EAC
- pain – usually only with acute infection

Features:
- narrowed canal – may be tender
- itching

- AIM = remove irritation factors and treat both infection and any underlying skin disorders

Initial Consultation

- Examine ear, if able to perform aural suction to remove residual debris, proceed with caution as the ear will be tender and may bleed.

- Take swab for culture and sensitivity

If the meatus is closed due to oedema, a ribbon gauze dressing soaked in Glycerine and Icthammol should be inserted to reduce the swelling and relieve inflammation. **Change dressing on alternate days** until meatus opens, if patient unable to attend or no clinic available a "POPE" wick soaked in Gentisone HC (if patient has no contraindications, see PGD) should be used and the patient advised to apply 3-4 drops 3 times daily directly onto wick for 7 days.

Review Patient 1 week

- Remove the debris and discharge with the suction, look for polyps, crusts and cholesteatoma.
- Review swab results.
- Local steroid and/or antibiotic drops should be dispensed according to the agreed protocol/PGD. This should be recorded in the patients notes.
- When inflammation settles the tympanic membrane should be examined for middle ear disease.

Review if unsure of findings

- ALWAYS document, date, time and sign findings, treatment and advice given
- Patients should be warned not to let water into their ears and not to use anything to scratch their ears (cotton buds, match sticks)

Review Patient in 2 weeks

- If condition resolved, given patient open appointment.
- If condition is still current, aural suction, review patient education, change medication if more than one sensitivity was given on swab report. Review as required for severity of condition, for chronic otitis externa this may be on a monthly basis. Each patient to be assessed individually.

POINTS TO REMEMBER

- a patient may develop an allergy to ear drops
- regular use of ear drops may precipitate a fungal infection
- patient to use the full course of medication
- Chronic Infection can be bacterial or fungal
- If unsure or condition fails to improve – refer
- record all findings and treatment given

GUIDELINES FOR THE TREATMENT OF MASTOID CAVITIES

TYPES OF MASTOID OPERATIONS

CORTICAL	performed to treat acute mastoiditis, surgical removal of the mastoid air cells leaving the ear canal and middle ear structures intact. Ear appears normal on examination and should self clean.
RADICAL	performed to control cholesteatoma, surgical removal of mastoid air cells, tympanic membrane, ossicles and middle ear mucosa, creating a single large cavity.
MODIFIED RADICAL	performed to control less extensive disease, tympanic membrane and ossicular chain preserved if possible.
ATTICOTOMY	performed to remove small attic cholesteatoma, ossicular chain intact, size and shape of cavity depends on extent of disease.
COMBINED APPROACH	endaural/postaural approach to remove TYMPANOPLASTY cholesteatoma avoiding destruction of hearing, often used in younger patients, appearance similar to cortical mastoidectomy.

Radical and some modified radical and atticotomies are unable to self clean and require regular aural toilet.

Cortical mastoidectomies and combined approach tympanoplasties require aural toilet and dewaxing if necessary. All crusts need to be removed because there may be active disease behind them.

1. CLEANING THE MASTOID CAVITY

- Position patient under the microscope
- Examine EAC, including meatal floor, the attic and posterior areas
- If cavity dry ⟶ review 6 – 12 months
- If cavity active ⟶ clean with microsuction
- Pearly, smelly mass or crusts indicates recurrence of Cholesteatoma ⟶ **REFER**
- Granular ⟶ TAC ointment, review 1 month, if unresolved ⟶ **REFER**
- If cavity discharging ⟶ clear debris with microsuction, Otomise for 2 weeks, review 1 month, if unresolved ⟶ **REFER**

2. REFERRAL

- Recurrence of cholesteatoma
- Chronically discharging cavity

GUIDELINES FOR THE TREATMENT OF FURUNCLE

A furuncle is a staphylococcal infection of the hair follicles found in the lateral part of the EAM. It presents with severe otalgia made worse by movement of the pinna and deafness. Examination is very difficult because of the pain. Most rupture spontaneously.

- Take a swab for culture and sensitivity

- Clean ear gently, this is a very painful condition

- Insert a Glycerine and Icthammol wick daily if possible, until inflammation is reduced (if not possible, change after 24 hours and then as clinics permit)

- REFER for systemic antibiotics and analgesia

- Explain to patient condition will get better, importance of compliance with treatment and advise to rest until pain subsides

GUIDELINES FOR REMOVAL OF FOREIGN BODIES

Most commonly found in children (beads, cotton wool buds etc). May be accompanied by discharge, bleeding, deafness and/or pain. Co-operation and a good light source are necessary, usually a child will allow only one attempt at removal which if unsuccessful will require a general anaesthetic, therefore, if you think you will be unable to remove the object easily refer to the doctor. If inserted deeply into the EAC a perforation of the tympanic membrane can result. Objects such as peas, peanuts and vegetable matter will swell if liquid is put into the ear making removal difficult.

AN OBJECT NEAR THE TYMPANIC MEMBRANE MUST BE REMOVED UNDER GENERAL ANAESTHETIC

1 Beads, stones and plastic objects

- Position patient under microscope
- Assess position in EAM
- REFER IF UNSURE
- Attempt removal with blunt hook or suction
- Assess tympanic membrane

INTACT ⟶ Discharge
PERFORATION ⟶ REFER
UNSUCCESSFUL ⟶ REFER

2 Soft objects

- Position patient under microscope
- Assess position of object in EAM
- REFER IN UNSURE
- Attempt removal with grasping forceps/suction
- Assess tympanic membrane

INTACT ⟶ Discharge
PERFORATION ⟶ REFER
UNSUCCESSFUL ⟶ REFER

3 Insects

- Position patient under microscope
- Assess position and status of insect in EAC
- REFER IF UNSURE
- If alive instil olive oil, alcohol or spirit to drown insect
- Attempt removal with suction or grasping forceps
- Assess tympanic membrane

INTACT ⟶ Discharge
PERFORATION ⟶ REFER
UNSUCCESSFUL ⟶ REFER

REFERRAL

- Failed attempt at removal
- Uncooperative child
- Suspected trauma to tympanic membrane
- Risk of damaging tympanic membrane during removal

GUIDELINES FOR THE MANUAL REMOVAL OF WAX

WAX

Ear Wax is a normal bodily secretion, it emerges from the external ear canal spontaneously, the skin from the lateral surface of the tympanic membrane is migratory travelling outwards from the ear drum and along the ear canal. Wax provides a protective film, therefore should only be removed if causing deafness, pain or it blocks the view of the tympanic membrane. Factors that prevent the normal extrusion of wax from the ear canal are wearing a hearing aid and patients attempting to clean their own ears with cotton buds. The wax is pushed deeper into the canal and compacted. Further attempts at removal can cause trauma and secondary otitis externa. Wax removal has been shown to improve hearing in-patients with impacted wax

Soft wax to be removed by aural suction – care must be taken not to traumatise the meatal wall.

- If the wax is too hard to remove wax softening agents are the first line of management. Trying to remove hard wax can tear the meatal skin allowing a portal of entry for infection.
- Sodium bicarbonate eardrops for 5 days, 3-4 drops to the affected ear twice daily. If the patient has perforation to tympanic membrane advise use of olive oil. Instructions as how to administer drops to be given to the patient.
- Review patients in 2 weeks

Examine ear to see if wax softened.

- When wax is removed check the tympanic membrane, examine the attic area.
- If any cholesteatoma, retraction pockets or perforations, document and refer to doctor if these are new findings.
- Document all observations, treatments (including rationale), information given to patient.
- Patients with chronic wax problem, advise to use olive oil on a prn basis to keep wax softer.
- Arrange follow up appointment or review.
- Send letter outlining changes to treatment to GP

Formal ENT-UK guidance for the use of aminoglycoside containing ear drops in the presence of a perforation

As published in Clinical Otolaryngology, Ref Phillips et al

Recommendation 1. The following items have to be adopted (as formal ENT-UK guidances) when treating a patient with a discharging ear, in whom there is a perforation or patent grommet.

1. If a topical aminoglycoside is used, this should only be in the presence of obvious infection.
2. Topical aminoglycosides should be used for no longer than 2 weeks.
3. The justification for using topical aminoglycosides should be explained to the patient.
4. Baseline audiometry should be performed, if possible or practical, before treatment with topical aminoglycosides.

Recommendation 2. ENT-UK should seek expert advice on the use of ototopical quinolones, specifically on the advisability of their un-licensed use for patients with a discharging ear, in whom there is a perforation or patent grommet. What are the potential adverse effects in terms of emergence of bacterial resistance?

Keypoints

- There seems to be little evidence linking vertigo or hearing loss to the short-term use of aminoglycoside-containing drops in discharging ears, in the presence of a grommet or perforation.
- The 'evidence' that does exist is of poor quality, consisting of data from a number of case reports and small case series.
- Prospective studies into the ototoxic effecs of aminoglycoside ear drops either support their use but lack power to statistically confirm this, or are preformed in conditions that are not representative of normal clinical conditions.
- Guidelines produced outside the UK recommend the use of quinolone containing drops that are not licensed in this country.
- Although it is possible for individual doctors to use such drops 'off license', it is appropriate that ENT-UK should issue guidance on the continued use of aminoglycoside-containing drops.
- Mindful of the need to produce clinical guidelines based on the best available evidence, the Clinical Audit and Practice Advisory Group of the British Association of Otolaryngologists – Head and Neck Surgeons (ENT-UK) has produced recommendations based on the views of an expert consensus panel.

EXAMPLE OF A PROTOCOL USED IN SOUTHPORT

PROTOCOL FOR THE ADMINISTRATION OF AURAL MEDICATIONS

MEDICATIONS FOR USE BY NURSES IN THE AURAL DRESSING CLINIC

OTOMIZE

Otitis externa
Chronic otitis externa
Chronic itching

LOCORTEN VIOFORM

Dry/flaky ears
Fungal infection

SOFRADEX

To clear out debris

GENTISONE HC

Otitis externa

The decision on which preparation to use depends on the severity of the Otitis Externa and the patient's manual dexterity.

- Care should be taken with antibiotic ear preparations because antibiotics can cause allergic skin reactions. They may also cause growth of secondary infections such as fungi and worsen the condition.
- To instil drops the head needs to be held with the ear uppermost and it is often easier for somebody else to put in the drops.
- Sprays are often easier for the patient to use themselves, and do not need specific positioning of the head. They do however need the ear canal to be fairly open.

Records must be kept of any patients experiencing adverse reactions and regular audit carried out.

Non response to treatment is often due to inadequate cleaning of the ear canal.

EXAMPLE OF THE PROTOCOL USED IN SOUTHPORT

GUIDELINES FOR AURAL MICROSUCTION

1) The Aural Dressing Clinic is staffed by a first level nurse who has completed a documented period of training under the supervision of an ENT Surgeon and/or aural care nurse practitioner of not less than six months.

2) Clinics take place in the ENT Out-Patient department.

3) Case records to be obtained, before treatment, for assessment of previous dressing clinic treatments and recording of any new treatments given.

4) All new patient referral letters are seen by a doctor and marked 'dressing clinic', the aural care nurse practitioner will assess priority for treatment and liaise with appointment staff and book patients accordingly.

5) All new patients will have an assessment record completed by the nurse practitioner on the patients initial visit, documenting past medical history, condition, symptoms and treatment.

6) Each follow up-appointment will be allocated a 20 minute appointment for discussion, treatment and documentation.

7) Verbal consent to treatment by a nurse to be obtained before any treatment.

8) Written guidelines for aural micro-suction must be adhered to.

9) Aural medications to be administered according to the agreed protocols. The nurse practitioner needs to complete a period of instruction and be signed competent by the ward manager, pharmacy and the ENT consultant as able to administer/dispense aural medication.

10) GP's to be informed by letter of their patients treatment and/or discharge from clinic.

11) Any patient refusing treatment, wishing to see a doctor or presenting with a condition beyond the nurse's remit must be given an appointment to see the next available doctor.

EXAMPLE OF AUDIT

SOUTHPORT AND FORMBY NHS TRUST
ENT OUTPATIENTS DEPARTMENT
AURAL MICRO SUCTION
YEARS 1992 – 1995

PERCENTAGE OF PATIENTS SEEN BY MEDICAL AND NURSING STAFF

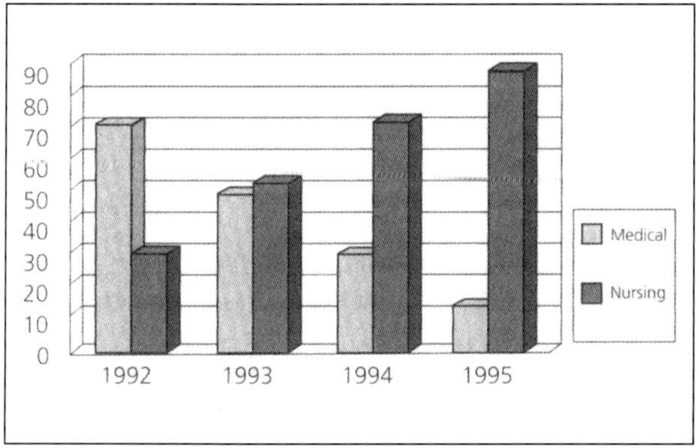

Chart demonstrating how the introduction of Nurse Microsuction causes decrease in patients needing to see a doctor from over 70% to 10%.

RANDOM RETROSPECTIVE AUDIT OF 50 PATIENTS WHO ATTENDED THE NURSE-LED AURAL DRESSING CLINIC DURING THE MONTHS OF SEPTEMBER AND OCTOBER, 2000

Variation Of Conditions

1	FOREIGN BODY	
19	WAX	3 UNILATERAL 16 BILATERAL
16	MASTOIDS	11 UNILATERAL 5 BILATERAL
12	OTITIS EXTERNA	
2	C.S.O.M	

Predisposing Factors For Removal of wax by Aural micro-suction.

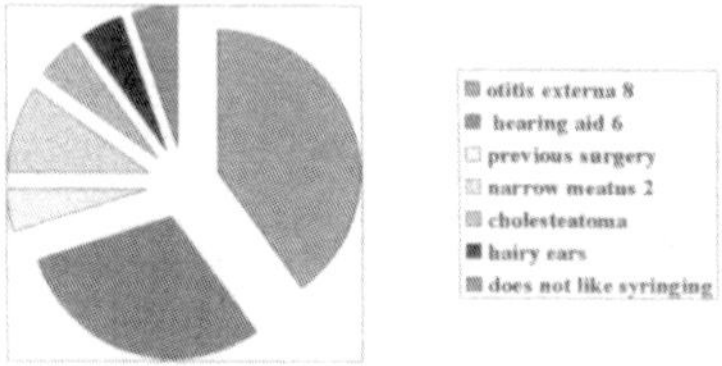

Mastoid Cavities

- 16 mastoid cavity clearances
- 11 patients had wax removed
- 5 patients treatment for discharging mastoid
- 4 patients had hearing aids – which contributed to their discharging ear

Otitis Externa predisposing factors

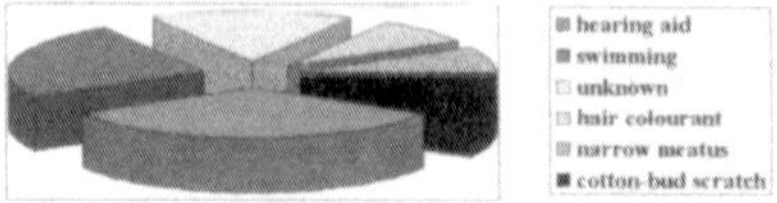

AURAL CARE CLINIC

Southport General Infirmary – Patient Attendance Figures
January 03 – December 03 Inclusive

Month	On clinic	Seen	Follow up	New	DNA	Canc
Jan	78	69	62	7	7	2
Feb	57	52	47	5	4	1
Mar	87	81	71	10	3	3
Apr	91	83	79	4	7	1
May	90	82	74	8	3	5
June	91	83	76	7	6	2
July	82	72	67	5	9	1
Aug	103	92	87	5	7	4
Sept	107	97	89	8	5	5
Oct	102	98	85	13	3	1
Nov	106	97	90	7	8	1
Dec	98	82	75	7	12	4
TOTAL	1092	988	902	86	74	30
Percent	100%	90%	91%	9%	7%	3%

1092 Patients booked on clinic
90% attendance (988 patients)

Of those attending
91% (902 patients) follow up patients seen
9% (86 patients) new patients seen

7% (74 patients) did not attend
3% (30 patients) cancelled

Patient attendance figures 2005

1204 patients booked on clinic
118 new patients (10%)
1086 follow ups (90%)

81 Patients did not attend in the year
Remaining a DNA rate of 7%

Suggested Training Program Based on the Training at Southport General Infirmary

AIM

To provide the nurse with the knowledge and practical skills to use microsuction in a safe, effective way.

Supervision

Consultant in charge of the department

Outcomes

1. Be able to describe the anatomy of a normal ear
2. Recognise abnormal anatomy
3. Understand basic ear conditions ie: otitis externa, wax, polyps, cholesteatoma
4. Perform safe microsuction
5. Understand the contraindications to microsuction
6. Be aware of the potential risks and when to refer for medical opinion

Part 1

Theoretical sessions to provide:

- anatomy and physiology
- clinical risk and accountability
- basic examination of ears
- ear diseases
- contra indications to microsuction

Part 2

- Period of observation of microsuction.
- Supervision of microsuction when nurse feels able (an agreed minimum number of cases needs to be established – for experienced ENT nurses this may be as little as 10 cases, see appendix)
- A record of all cases seen and treated must be kept by the nurse

Part 3

- Assessment of competence:
  Independent treatment of an agreed number of cases checked by the Consultant

SUGGESTED EQUIPMENT REQUIRED TO SET UP AURAL CARE CLINIC

ENT MICROSCOPE WITH TEACHING ARM ATTACHMENT 250mm LENS

ADJUSTABLE HI/LO EXAMINATION COUCH

ADJUSTABLE HEIGHT STOOL

1 SUCTION MACHINE, BOTTLE AND LENGTHS OF FLEXIBLE TUBING

MAYO TROLLEY OR DRESSING TROLLEY

SUITABLE CLINIC ROOM

Range of Instruments

AURAL SPECULUM (OBLIQUE ENDED)

SET OF 5 IN VARYING SIZES

INDIVIDUAL SIZES	NO 3 NO 4 NO 5

ZOELLNER SUCTION TUBES

ST. BARTS MODEL BLUNT WAX HOOK

JOBSON HORNE PROBES (5½" LENGTH)

TILLEY AURAL DRESSING FORCEPS

HARTMANNS AURAL FORCEPS (CROCODILE, SERRATED EDGE) 2 SIZES

STORAGE FACILITIES FOR INSTRUMENTS.

Supplementaries

ZOELLNER FINE ENDS 18SWG

AURAL SWABS

2ML SYRINGES

MEDIPLAST METAL TIPS APPLICATOR ENDS

STERILE RIBBON GAUZE (1.25CM WIDE)

POPE OTO WICKS

GALLIPOTS

TISSUES

STERILE WATER

STERILE COTTON WOOL

RECEIVERS

GLOVES

CASE STUDIES

Case Study 1

A 25 year old man complains of acute right ear pain. He also noticed a watery discharge from the ear. He has recently returned from holiday abroad.

Symptoms

Pronounced ear pain; decreased hearing in the right ear; and a thin watery discharge are present. Onset of symptoms occurred 5 days ago and have been progressively worsening.

Relevant patient history

No history of allergies or acute otitis media. He has no OE history, but admitted to swimming daily whilst on holiday.

Physical findings

The patient exhibits guarding of the right ear and complains of tenderness when the tragus is manipulated during the examination. The ear canal appears severely inflamed, occluding the lumen of the canal. Little erythema is present. Swelling makes visualization of the tympanic membrane impossible.

Diagnosis

Diffuse acute bacterial OE.

Treatment

1. Gently clean the discharge from the ear canal and take a swab for culture and sensitivity.
2. Insert Glycerine & Ichthammol wick.
3. Advise on analgesics
4. Return in 24 hours and then provide antibiotic steroid drops eg, Neomycin plus Betnesol or, when they become available in the UK, a Fluroquinolone & steroid combination.

It may be beneficial to insert a wick to ensure delivery of medication because of the degree of inflammation in this patients ear canal.

Discussion

Use of the Aminoglycoside or Fluoroquinolones provides excellent coverage of the pathogens most frequently associated with OE. Unlike the Aminoglycoside-containing preparations, the Fluoroquinolones are not associated with any ototoxicity. The steroid component offers an additional benefit because it helps relieve inflammation and provides quicker resolution of pain.

Follow up

Advise patient regarding proper administration of the medication and address the importance of finishing the course of therapy even if the symptoms resolve. Instruct the patient to return again if the condition does not improve or if it worsens.

Case Study 2

A 69 year old woman presents with complaints of unresolved bacterial OE involving the left ear. Despite a 10 day course of therapy with Ear Calm, (Hydrocortisone and Ascetic Acid Otic solution) the infection has not resolved.

Symptoms

Intense pain in the left ear, some loss of hearing, continued discharge,

Relevant patient history

In addition to the OE, the patient has a history of diabetes mellitus

Physical findings

Examination of the ear reveals inflammation of the canal and some erythema.

Diagnosis

A diagnosis of malignant OE is made on the basis of the clinical findings and confirmed by the bone scan.

Treatment

Therapy is immediately instituted with a systemic antibiotic agent such as Ciprofloxacin with topical aminoglycoside antibiotic treatment.

Discussion

Several years ago the mortality associated with malignant OE was as high as 80%. Today, with the development of improved treatment modalities, the mortality has decreased to 3-4%. Combination oral and topical treatment is necessary to halt the progression of the infection. It is prudent to treat any diabetic patient with acute OE with a combination of topical and systemic antibiotic agents. If the patients appears toxic or has a cranial nerve palsy, then initial therapy with intravenous antibiotics in addition to topical agents should be employed.

Case Study 3

A 14 year old girl returns to the clinic with itching and discharge of the left ear. She complains of having a "blocked up" ear.

Physical findings

Examination of the left ear reveals a thin, watery discharge and inflammation of the EAC. Hearing reduction is noted.

Relevant Patient History

The patient, a swimmer on the local school team, has a history of recurrent OE. Three days ago she had been diagnosed with acute OE and was prescribed Sofradex (Soframycin and Polymyxin B and Dexamethasone).

Diagnosis

Acute OE but possibly a topical reaction to Soframycin

Therapeutic intervention

Patient is advised to immediately discontinue use of Soframycin and an analgesic for pain relief. Glycerine & Ichthammol wick was inserted. If the condition is severe, occasionally systemic steroid may be warranted.

Discussion

Amino glycoside reactions are common (up to 1/3 of patients are affected) and can range from mild to severe. Patients will be advised to discontinue use of this agent. Additional medication will be prescribed (eg Fluoroquinolones, analgesics), and follow-up visits to the doctor are warranted.

Follow up

The patient is shown the proper administration techniques and is instructed to take the medication as prescribed. She is also told to call if the condition does not improve. If seborrhea or eczema are present at this time, then the patient should be treated with 2.% Hydrocortisone cream. The cream should be used twice a day until the itching and flaking resolve and then twice a week for prophylaxis, as this agent may reduce the likelihood of recurrent OE.

But most importantly she should use fitted ear plugs held in by a bathing cap when swimming or change sport.

Southport & Ormskirk Hospital NHS Trust

Patient group direction for the supply/administration of Gentisone HC ear drops for the treatment of otitis externa and discharging mastoid cavities in the aural care clinics.

Directorate/Department	Surgical – ENT
Statement	The staff in the staff group may administer/supply without medical prescription as detailed in this document
Staff group	Nurse practitioners in aural care clinics
Situation/condition	New and follow up patients attending nurse-led aural care clinic presenting with: • Otitis externa • Prophylaxis against otitis externa following trauma • Mastoid cavities
Inclusion	• Over 16 years • In response to swab results (sensitivities) • To be used in the presence of a perforated tympanic membrane, only if systemic antibiotics have failed to settle infection, or the doctor has documented use of treatment in patients case notes.
Exclusion	• Children under 16 • Pregnancy or thinking of becoming pregnant • Allergy to Gentamicin or other components • Perforated tympanic membrane – refer to doctor on initial treatment • No active infection • Culture and sensitivity from recent ear swab does not recommend spray • If fungal infection is suspected
Action if included	Supply drops only after thorough clinic of the external auditory canal. Apply with gauze/Oto-wicks which are kept saturated with eardrops for the treatment of severe otitis externa.
Action if excluded or non compliant	Refer to see doctor
Name of Medicine	Gentisone HC ear drops
POM/P/GSL	POM
Dose	Three drops
Route/method	Application to external auditory canal

Frequency	3 times daily for 5-7 days	
Total dose/number	Up to a maximum of 3 courses	
Information on follow up treatment	As per guidelines for otitis externa and mastoid cavities	
Written/verbal advice for patient care before/after treatment	• Educate patient as recommendations for otitis externa/ear care advice – give leaflet • Advise on how to administer drops • Advise that some stinging may be experienced for the first few days of treatment • Advise that once bottle opened not to be used after 1 month of opening	
Adverse drug reaction and management	Inform patient if experiences excess pain, itching inflammation whilst on treatment to contact department and discontinue treatment. Appointment to be given for the next aural care clinic.	
Specify method of recording sufficient to include audit	The date, drug name and batch number HC form issue of medication form	
Protocol approved by	**Name**	**Signature**
Author:		
Reviewing pharmacist:		
Consultant clinician:		
Non medical prescribing Lead:		
Senior Pharmacist:		
Chairman of Drug and Therapeutic Committee:		
Clinical Governance Lead:		
Consultant Microbiologist: (if appropriate)		
Nurse/AHP:		
Version		
Date approved .... **Review Date** .... **(+2 years)**		

Southport & Ormskirk Hospital NHS Trust

Patient group direction for the supply/administration of Otomise ear spray for the treatment of otitis externa and discharging mastoid cavitiets in the aural care clinics

Directorate/Department	Surgical – ENT
Statement	The staff in the staff group may administer/supply without medical prescription as detailed in this document
Staff group	Nurse practitioners in aural care clinics
Situation/condition	New and follow up patients attending nurse-led aural care clinic presenting with: • **Otitis externa** • **Mastoid cavities**
Inclusion	• Over 16 years • In response to swab results (sensitivities) • To be used in the presence of a perforated tympanic membrane, only if systemic antibiotics have failed to settle infection, or the doctor has documented use of treatment in patients case notes.
Exclusion	• Children under 16 • Pregnancy or thinking of becoming pregnant • Allergy to Neomycin or other components • Perforated tympanic membrane – refer to doctor on initial treatment • No active infection • Culture and sensitivity from recent ear swab does not recommend spray • If fungal infection is suspected
Action if included	Supply spray only after thorough cleaning of the external auditory canal Document in patients case notes and issue of Otomise form
Action if excluded or non compliant	Refer to see doctor
Name of Medicine	**Otomise ear drops**
POM/P/GSL	POM
Dose	One spray
Route/method	Ear spray for application to external auditory canal
Frequency	3 times daily for 5-7 days

Total dose/number	Up to a maximum of 3 courses	
Information on follow up treatment	As per guidelines for otitis externa and mastoid cavities	
Written/verbal advice for patient care before/after treatment	• Educate patient as recommendations for otitis externa/ear care advice – give leaflet • Advise on how to administer spray • Advise that some stinging may be experienced for the first few days of treatment • Advise that once bottle opened not to be used after 1 month of opening	
Adverse drug reaction and management Specify method of recording sufficient to include audit	Inform patient if experiences excess pain, itching inflammation whilst on treatment to contact department and discontinue treatment. Appointment to be given for the next aural care clinic. The date, drug name and batch number will be recorded on the case notes. An issue of medication form will be completed for re-stock	
Protocol approved by	**Name**	**Signature**
Author:		
Reviewing pharmacist:		
Consultant clinician:		
Non medical prescribing Lead:		
Senior Pharmacist:		
Chairman of Drug and Therapeutic Committee:		
Clinical Governance Lead:		
Consultant Microbiologist: (if appropriate)		
Nurse/AHP:		
Version 1		

Date approved .... **Review Date** .... **(+2 years)**

TABLE FOR TRAINING

Conditions Observed

Date	Type of Condition being Treated	Signature of Supervising Consultant / Nurse Trainer	Reflection

Aural Microsuction Carried out by Trainee Under Direct Supervision with Trainer Observing

Date	Type of Condition being Treated	Signature of Supervising Consultant / Nurse Trainer	Reflection

Aural Microsuction With Patient Examined and Interview by Trainer after the Procedure has been Undertaken

Date	Type of Condition being Treated	Observation & Signature of Supervising Consultant / Nurse Trainer

Suggested Reading

Bull P. D.	Diseases of the Ear, Nose and Throat. Blackwell Science. Oxford. 1996
Ali-Raza S, Denholm S. W, Wong J. C. H.	An audit of the management of acute otitis externa in an ENT casualty clinic Journal of Laryngology and Otology 1995; 109: 130-133
England R. J. A, Homer J. J, Jasser P, Wilde A. D.	Accuracy of patient self-medication with topical ear drops Journal of Laryngology and Otology 2000; 114: 24-25
Nilssen E, Wormald P. J, Oliver S.	Glycerol and icthammol: medicinal solution or mythical potion? Journal of Laryngology and Otology 1996; 110: 319-321
Roland N.J, McRae R.D.R, McCombe A.W.	Key Topics in Otolaryngology. 2nd ed. BIOS Scientific. Oxford. 2001
Russell J. D, Donnelly M, McShane D. P, Alun-Jones T, Walsh M.	What causes acute otitis externa? Journal of Laryngology and Otology 1993; 107: 898-901
Wormald P.J and Browning G.G.	Otoscopy a structured approach. Arnold. London. 1996
Wilde A.D, England J, Jones A. S.	An alternative to regular dressings for otitis externa and chronic supperative otitis media. Journal of Laryngology and Otology 1995; 109: 101-103
Zeitoun H.	Developing a nurse-led aural care clinic. Nursing Times 1997; 45: 46-47

References

Bapat U, Nia Bance M, (2001)
Severe audio-vestibular loss following ear syringing for wax removal
In: **The journal of Laryngology and Otology**
May 2001. Vol. 155. Pg 410-411

Blake P, Matthews R, Homibrook J (1998)
When not to syringe an ear
In: **New Zealand Medical Journal**
13th November 1998. Pg 422-424

B.N.F 44 Sept 2002
B.N.F Organisation

Browning G (2001)
Wax in the ear – Ear Nose and Throat Disorders
In: **Clinical evidence (2002)**
British Medical Journal, Publishing Group London

Dinsdale R (1991)
Catastrophic Otological Injury from Oral Jet Irrigation of the External Auditory Canal.
In: **Laryngoscope** 1991. Vol. 101. Pg 75-78

Eekhof JAH, De Bock GH, Le Cessie, S, Springer MP (2001)
A quasi-randomised controlled trial of water as a quick softening agent of persistent earwax in general practice.
In: **British Journal of General Practice**
2001. Vol. 51. Pg 635-637

Fahmy S, Whitfield H (1982)
Multi-Centre clinical trial of Exterol as a cerumenolytic
In: **British Journal of Clinical Practice**
1982. Vol. 36. Pg 197-204

Grossan M (1998)
Cerumen removal – current challenges
In: **Ear, nose and Throat Journal**
July 1998. Vol 77. No 7. Pg 541-548

Hawke M (2002)
Update on cerumen and ceruminolytics
In: www.entjournal.com/html/article-11-0208.html

Kent MA (1998)
The rationale behind the selection of ear syringing equipment
In: **British Journal of Community Nursing**
1998. Vol. 3. No 8. Pg 398-404

Medical Devices Agency (1998)
Safety Notice ear irrigator (pulsed water syringe) Propulse"
In: **SN (1998) 07** London Medical Devices Agency

Memel D, Langley C, Watkins C, Laue B, Birchall M, Bachmann M, (2002)
Effectiveness of ear syringing in general practice: a randomised controlled trial and patients experiences.
In: **British Journal of General Practice**
November 2002. Vol. 52. Pg 906-911

NHS Modernisation Agency
Action on ENT Good Practice Guide (October 2002)
Department of Health, Crown copyright

Price J (1997)
Problems of ear syringing
In: **Practice Nurse** 1997. Vol. 14. No. 2. Pg 126-128

Sharp, JF, Wilson JA, Ross L, Barr-Hamilton RH, (1990)
Ear wax removal: A survey of current practice
In: **British Medical Journal** 1990. Vol. 301. Pg 1251-1252

Vibeke Z, Sorensen MD, Per Bonding MD (1995)
Can ear irrigation cause rupture of the normal tympanic membrane? an experimental study in man.
In: **Journal of Laryngology and Otology**
Nov, 1995. Vol. 109. Pg 1036-1040

Phillips J.S et al (2007)
Evidence review and ENT-UK consensus report for the use of aminoglycoside-containing ear drops in the presence of an open middle ear.
In: **Clinical Otolaryngology**
October 2007. Vol. 32. No. 5. Pg 330-336

MANAGEMENT OF EARACHE

ONSET ← **PAIN** → **MORE THAN 24 HOURS**

ONSET → Use Paracetamol for 24 hours, withhold antibiotics at this stage

Immunoglobins Within exudates on the middle ear, may well cope with the infection

MORE THAN 24 HOURS → Treat likely bacterial otitis media with appropriate anticiotics

→ **REVIEW** ←

In two weeks to exclude secretory otitis media (glue ear)

- Earache with History of under-lying ear discharge
- Secretory otitis causing persistent deafness
- Recurrent acute otitis media causing patental or GP concern
- Earache complicated by ear discharge

→ **REFER** ←

If there is a history of previous ear surgery on discharging ear, or evidence of any surgical scarring around the ear, a detailed examination is required.

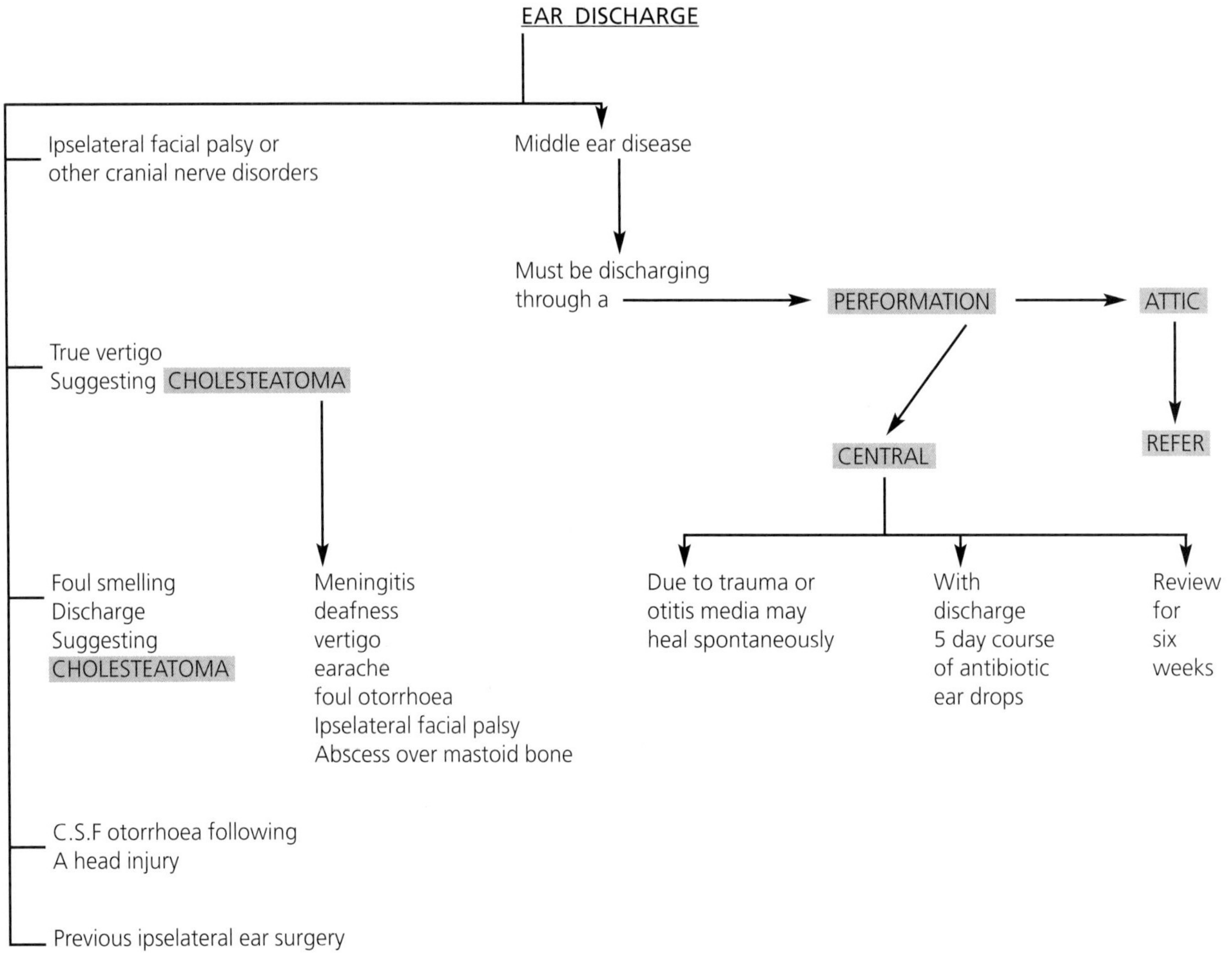
EAR DISCHARGE
Ipselateral facial palsy or other cranial nerve disorders
Middle ear disease
Must be discharging through a
PERFORMATION
ATTIC
REFER
CENTRAL
True vertigo
Suggesting CHOLESTEATOMA
Foul smelling
Discharge
Suggesting
CHOLESTEATOMA
Meningitis
deafness
vertigo
earache
foul otorrhoea
Ipselateral facial palsy
Abscess over mastoid bone
Due to trauma or otitis media may heal spontaneously
With discharge 5 day course of antibiotic ear drops
Review for six weeks
C.S.F otorrhoea following
A head injury
Previous ipselateral ear surgery

OTITIS EXTERNA

Eczematous condition of the external canal± causing itch, pain and moisture usually occurs

UNILATERAL

Cases are usually secondary to:

- Pseudomonas – swab to exclude pseudomonas. Usually in diabetics. Condition can be severely erosive. If so: → **REFER**
- Trauma eg. foreign body or hearing aid friction → **REFER**
- Furuncle, very painful **REFER** Acutely for in-patient Management
- Malignancy – very rarely

BILATERAL

TREATMENT

- Initial treatment with antibiotic steroid compound drops for 5 days
- Advise on avoidance of shampoo, swimming, bath water
- If patient is diabetic swab to exclude pseudomonas. If so **REFER**

IF THESE FAIL, REPEAT OTOSCOPY

Narrow canals with swollen walls → Treat with Glycerine/ ichthammol ribbon gauze 3 x week for 2 weeks → Resolution

- Canal still swollen **REFER**
- Canal open but debris still present

Treat with ½" ribbon gauze in-situ for 5 days with antibotic installation onto gauze 3 x day

- Persistent debris → **REFER**
- Debris removed leaving inflamed wall, use drops for further 5 days without gauze. if this does not settle → **REFER**

Aural Care and Microsuction in the Community with service maintenance

A model of rotation of skilled Nurses in Aural Care and Microsuction between Primary and secondary care. The benefits of this model provide a core group of highly skilled Nurses who would provide Aural Care and Microsuction for patients at a location near to where they live. CPD and training and supervision is delivered by a Consultant ENT Surgeon in Secondary care.

Aural Care Community/Hospital Axis

- 8 nurses of whom all should be Post Aural Care Course. E.g. Rotherham, Blackburn, Southport and Aintree
- Nurses A, B, C, D, E, F, G and H each working 4 sessions per week in Aural Care. 1 and ½ in hospital and 2 and ½ in Community Clinics. This is 10 hospital sessions per week and 20 Community sessions
- 1 consultant session per week to supervise Wednesday mornings
- Wednesday a.m. 9-10.30 Clinic 7. Difficult cases, teaching, audit and update A,B,C and D alternate weeks and E,F,G and H alternate weeks

Hospital sessions

Nurses work in pairs to cover sick leave and cross cover holidays between pairs.
9 patients per nurse new and old. 20 mins per patient when working at full stretch.

Monday	A+B
Tuesday	C+D
Wednesday	A+B+C+D alt weeks and E+F+G+H alt weeks
Thursday	E+F
Friday	G+H

Community sessions

Nurses work in pairs to cover sick leave and cross cover holidays between pairs.
9 patients per nurse new and old. 20 mins per patient when working at full stretch.

Monday	C+D+G+H
Tuesday	A+B+E+F
Wednesday	E+F+G+H alt weeks and A+B+C+D alt weeks
Thursday	G+H+C+D
Friday	E+F+A+B

Notes

Notes

Notes